THE
Tasmania Pantry Cookbook

Simple and delicious recipes inspired by Tasmanian growers and producers

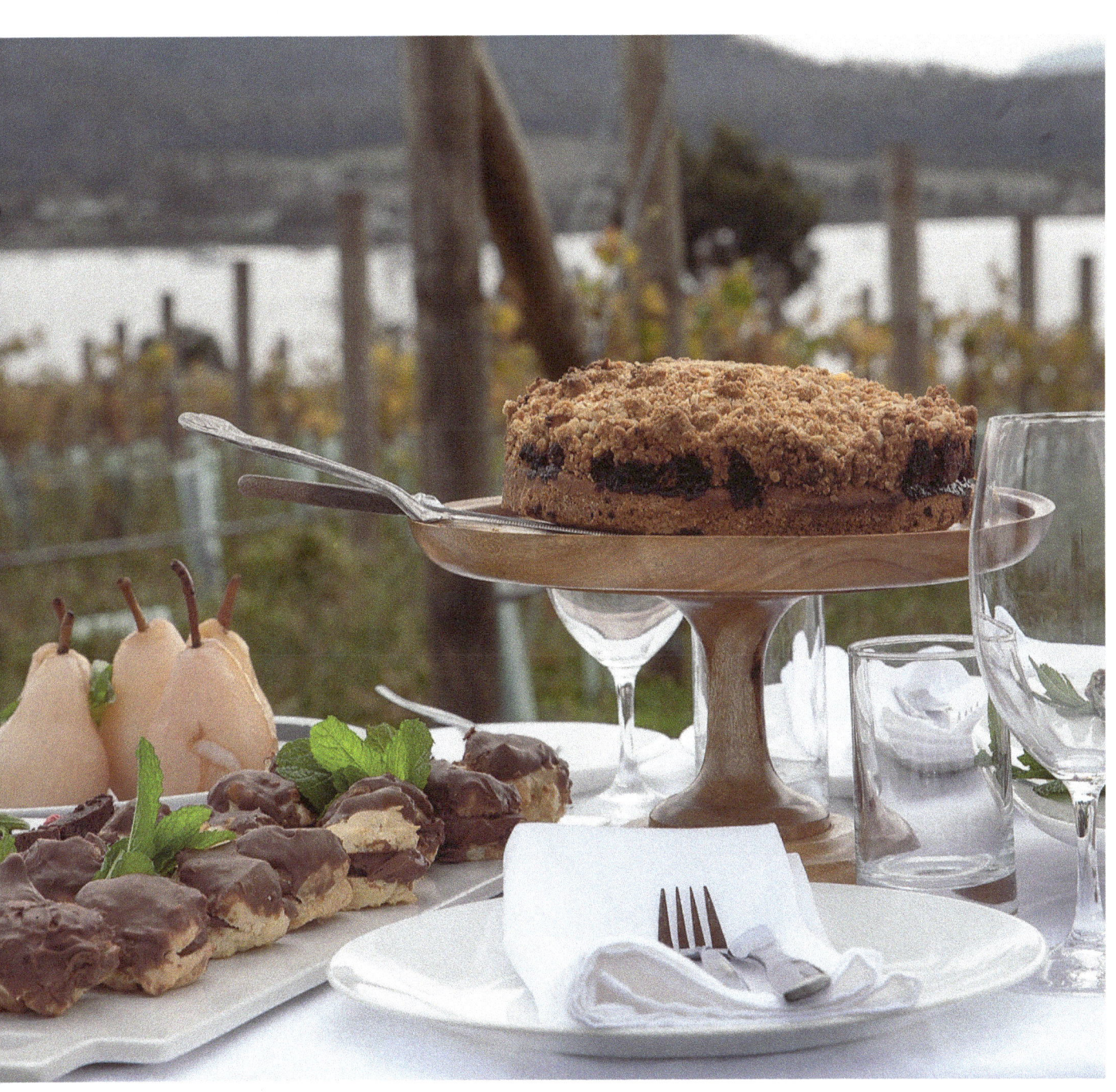

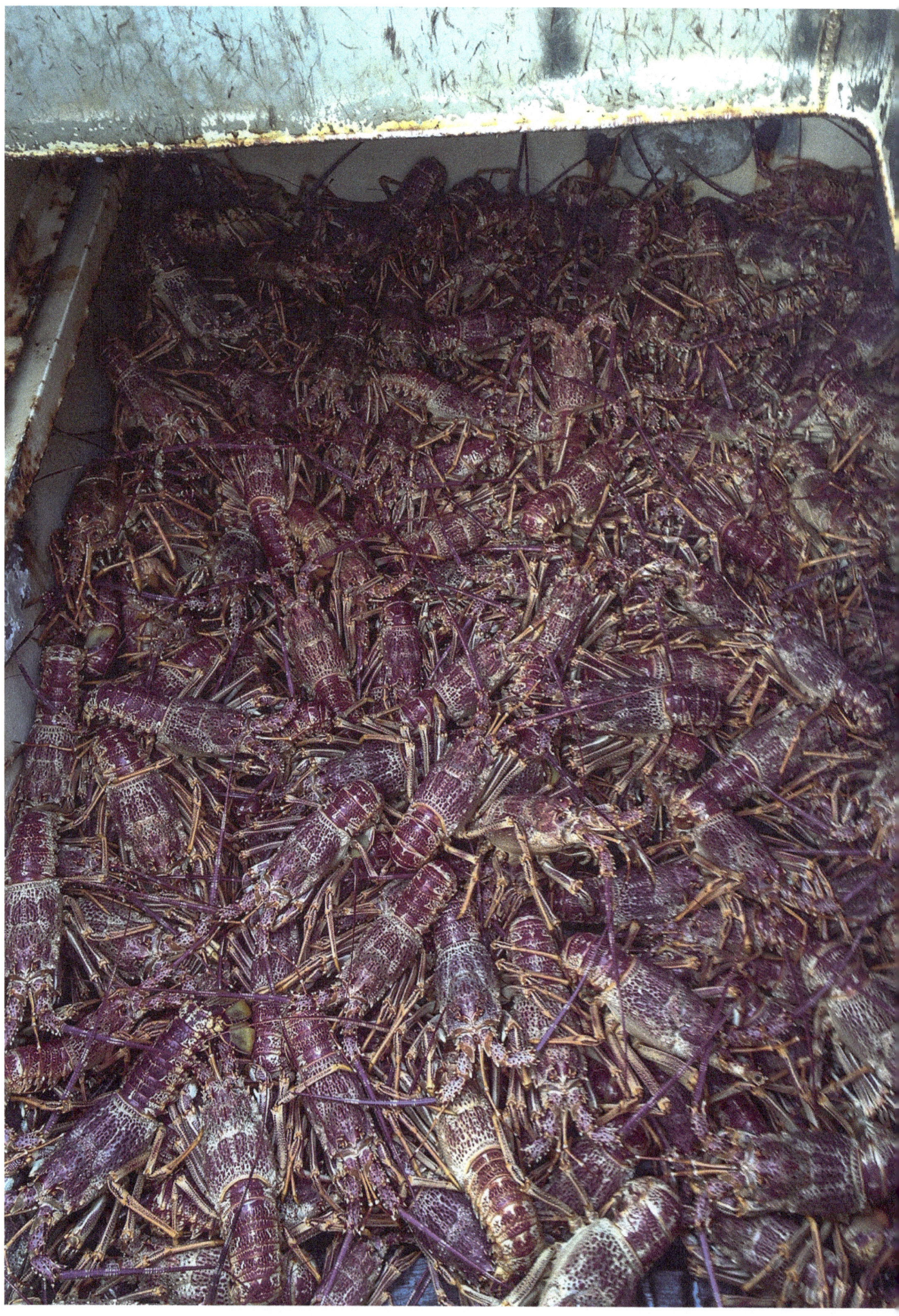

The Tasmanian Pantry Cookbook

Living in Tasmania, we are so lucky to be connected to our food. I had a wonderful childhood in the country, and today my own children spend loads of time in the country too - either around our home on the Tasman Peninsula or at the family shack on Bruny Island. I remember my Dad bringing home buckets of fresh fish and seafood and chasing the (slightly scared!) kids around with a crayfish. We picked or pinched apples from the orchard next-door, and hoped to not get caught by the farmer! I remember the stench of mutton birds slow cooking for days and running around green fields collecting giant mushrooms. We would wake up in the morning at our family shack to see uncle Paul had left a row of skinned wallabies, hanging up on the clothesline. I still remember Aunty Julie with a simply enormous bag of baby onions to pickle, and I have not so fond memories of my Mum's rabbit stew and the fun, and pain, we endured blackberry picking all summer. All these experiences added up to me having a real love of real, high quality food. I love to know where it comes from, and I love to eat it!

We now have a health crisis with obesity. This puts a strain on the heath system and is frustratingly preventable. I am happy to admit that I am a packet food snob. Although sugar, salt and fat each have a place in a healthy diet, these are also natural preservatives - so any packet food will have an excess of one, or all three of these to preserve it - even when it is labelled 'healthy' or 'natural'! I think packet food is for convenience, and is for occasional use. But rows and rows of "healthy packet food" appear in the supermarket these days, convincing us that we are too busy to find the time to prepare a meal. I also think the argument of commercialised fast food chains being a cheap place for a family meal is completely wrong – I could pick up a prime cut of meat at my local farmer's market, along with locally grown veggies, for the same price as a family meal at a fast food restaurant, and cook a beautiful, healthy meal for my family instead. Any qualified nutritionist will tell you our diets should be made up of mostly fresh vegetables, with fruit and protein and whole grains, and once you are organised with these products in your pantry - it really is easy. I am shocked and saddened when a teenager working in a supermarket asks me what a cauliflower is because he cannot identify it or look up the button on the till. I'm bored and sick of hearing about the latest elimination diet. Diets don't work, ever! Furthermore, some of those diets endorsed by celebrities are dangerous and then push the price of certain foods that should be accessible to everyone, sky high!

Weight loss if required is only achievable through expending more calories than you consume and eating the correct nutrients. Sometimes checking in and calorie counting is a good thing for all of us, as it makes you think twice before handing a packet of biscuits to the kids to keep them quiet at after school activities! But I want my kids to have a good relationship with food. The best parenting advice I ever read was to provide my children with 3 healthy meals and 2 healthy snacks - and they WILL eat. It works, and it is simple. They won't starve themselves, but they also probably won't eat their veggie sticks if there's a biscuit on offer instead! Children won't eat dinner if they are full of snacks either. Good delicious home cooked food can be healthy. Good health and good, delicious food can co-exist.

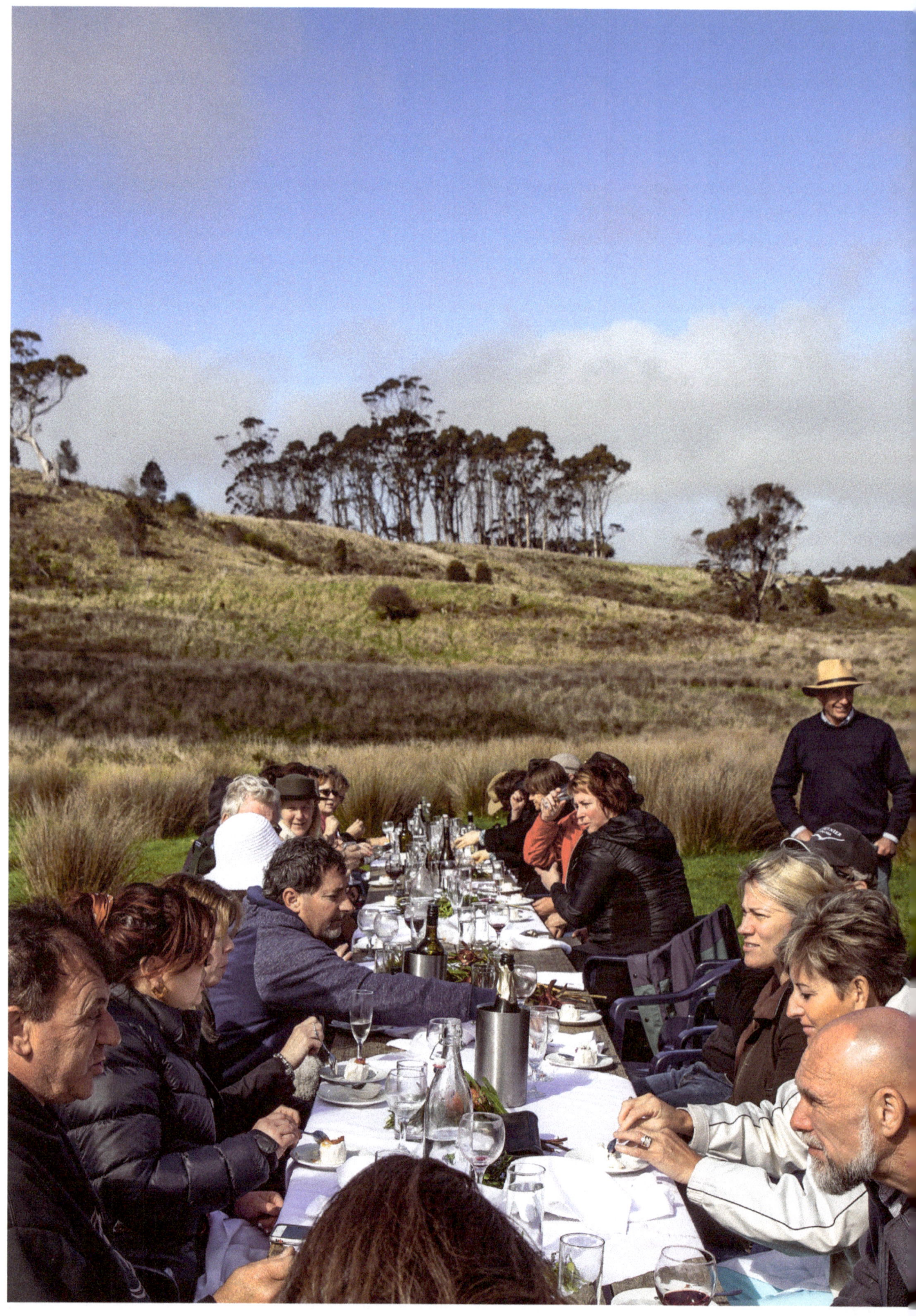

Cooking your food, proper old-fashioned meal planning and knowing what is in your food really it is the only healthy diet – and this should be coupled with a healthy active lifestyle. For example, carbohydrates are not the devil. If you eat porridge for breakfast, sushi for lunch and pasta for dinner, and you're putting on weight, carbs are not the problem - all three of these meals are perfectly healthy in a balanced diet, but it is just poor meal planning to blame. When did we get too busy to cook? When did we get too busy to plan our meals properly? Shouldn't feeding our family properly be a priority? When did buying a jar full of sugar & salt called easy tomato pasta sauce become SO MUCH easier than quickly chopping a onion and garlic and some actual tomatoes? When you think about it it's not really easier...at all. So I'm not claiming that the recipes in this book are all health food. As much as I would love to, we don't eat butter chicken and black forest trifle every night, but we do enjoy them occasionally. I certainly don't put toffee apples in the school lunch box but we do love making them a few times a year as a fun family activity, because after all, food is also for pleasure. I believe in all things in moderation - I certainly love a glass of wine so I am not going to stop my kids having the occasional treat. If they have the occasional soft drink I try to make sure it comes from a boutique family producer and they now prefer these choices.

You know what else? Cooking can be actually enjoyable and not a chore. If you hate cooking, why not try and change your mindset? Plan your meals, feel proud that you are feeding your family properly and feel happy when you support a local business. I don't want my kids to have a fear of food but if they are having a treat I would much prefer it to be something they have prepared with love, or being involved in it's preparation – whether it's picking strawberries to make the jam for Monte Carlo biscuits or making toffee apples.

This book is a collaboration of recipes supplied by chefs and suppliers around Tasmania, for you to cook in your home, hopefully, with good friends and delicious Tasmanian wine or beverage! I hope you enjoy.

Eloise Emmett

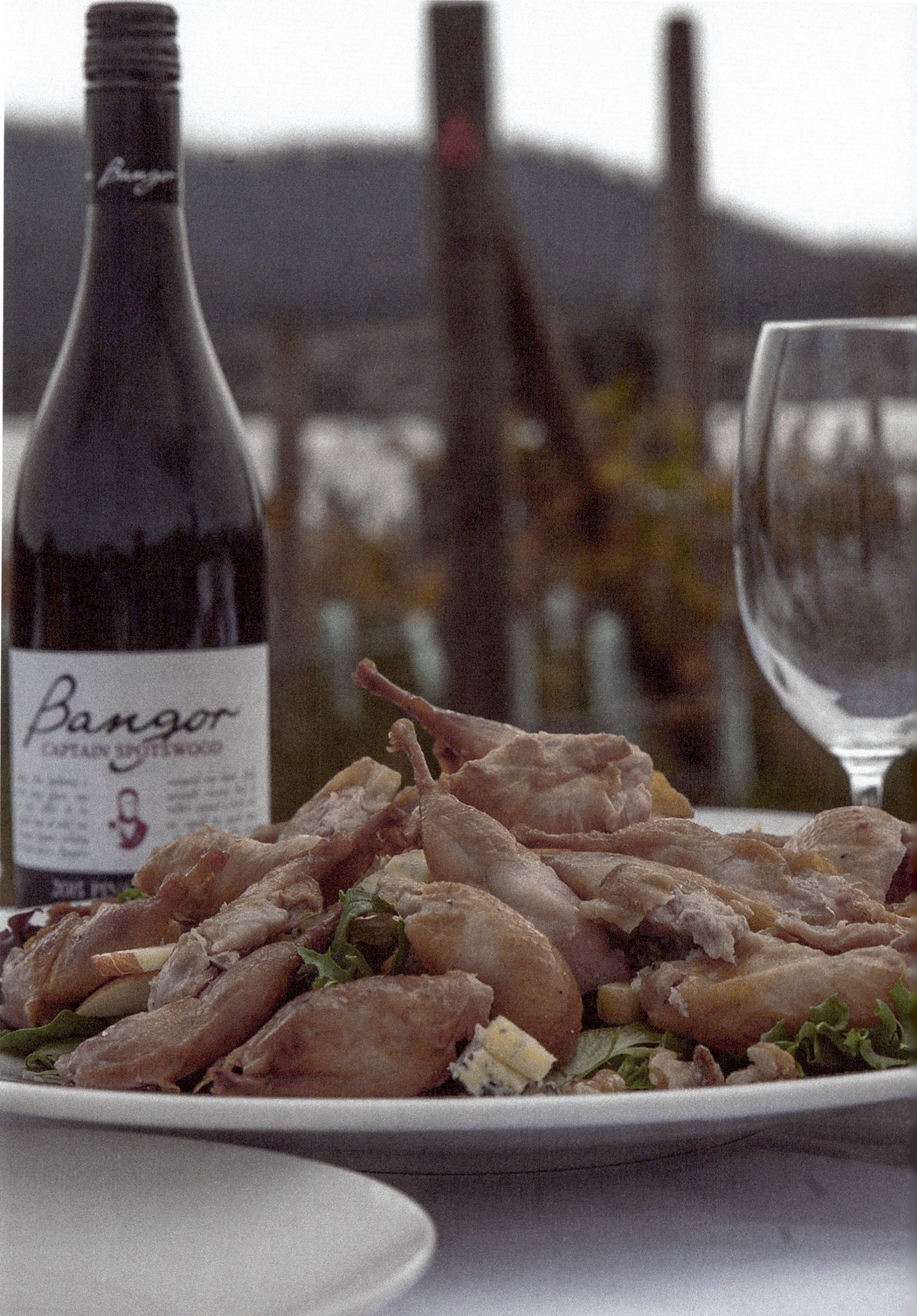

Acknowledgements

Thanks to all the readers of eloiseemmett.com and Instagram and Facebook followers who inspire me to create new recipes regularly.

Thanks to my workshop, event and dinner guests at Little Norfolk Bay Events and Chalets, who taste all the recipes and inspire me to create new dishes.

Thanks to my family, my husband Brendan and children Maggie, Stephanie and Oscar who are happy to pop on a good shirt for a photo and enjoy all the foods.

Thanks to Kylie Berry, Stokely 9 Design, for the beautiful design and support with the creation of this book.

Thanks to Arwen Genge for helping with the cooking for the recipe photos..

Thank you to Katharine Burke for adding her lovely words to the recipes and Sarah Carless and Bernie Carr for editing the book.

And a big thanks to all the sponsors and recipe contributors that have made this book possible and who have been so helpful, encouraging and enthusiastic to work with on this project:

- Kate Field
- Ana Pimento
- Damien Viney
- Anne Ashbolt
- Jess Doolan and Caroline Housel
- Suzanne Macefield
- Bernice and Richard Woolley
- Phil Lamb
- Anne McVilly, Sarah Morse, Mel Copping & Jennifer Fitzpatrick
- Clare Dean
- Kate Field
- Vanessa Dunbabin
- Peter and Nick Derkly
- Matt Rao
- Abby Mckibben
- Rebbecca Sims and Tracy Martin
- Susan Catchpole
- Penni Lampry
- Arwen Genge
- Grace Nieuwenhuizen
- Sharee Mills
- Steven Lund
- Matthew Dudman
- Chexi

- Leap Farm
- Meat Your Beef Farm Tours, King Island
- Spreyton Cider
- Ashbolt Farm
- Tassal
- Get Shucked Oysters
- Bruny Island Wines Bar and Grill
- Spring Bay Mussels
- Port Arthur Historic Site
- Port Arthur Lavender Farm
- Tongola Dairy Products
- Bangor Farm
- Lufra Hotel and Apartments
- The Italian Pantry
- Huon Aquaculture
- Petuna Seafoods
- Rockwall Bar and Grill
- Bee Patient Honey
- Arwen's Thermo Pics
- Made in Marion
- Endless Waves Hairdressing
- Chefaholic Cooking School
- Tassal
- Brockley Estate

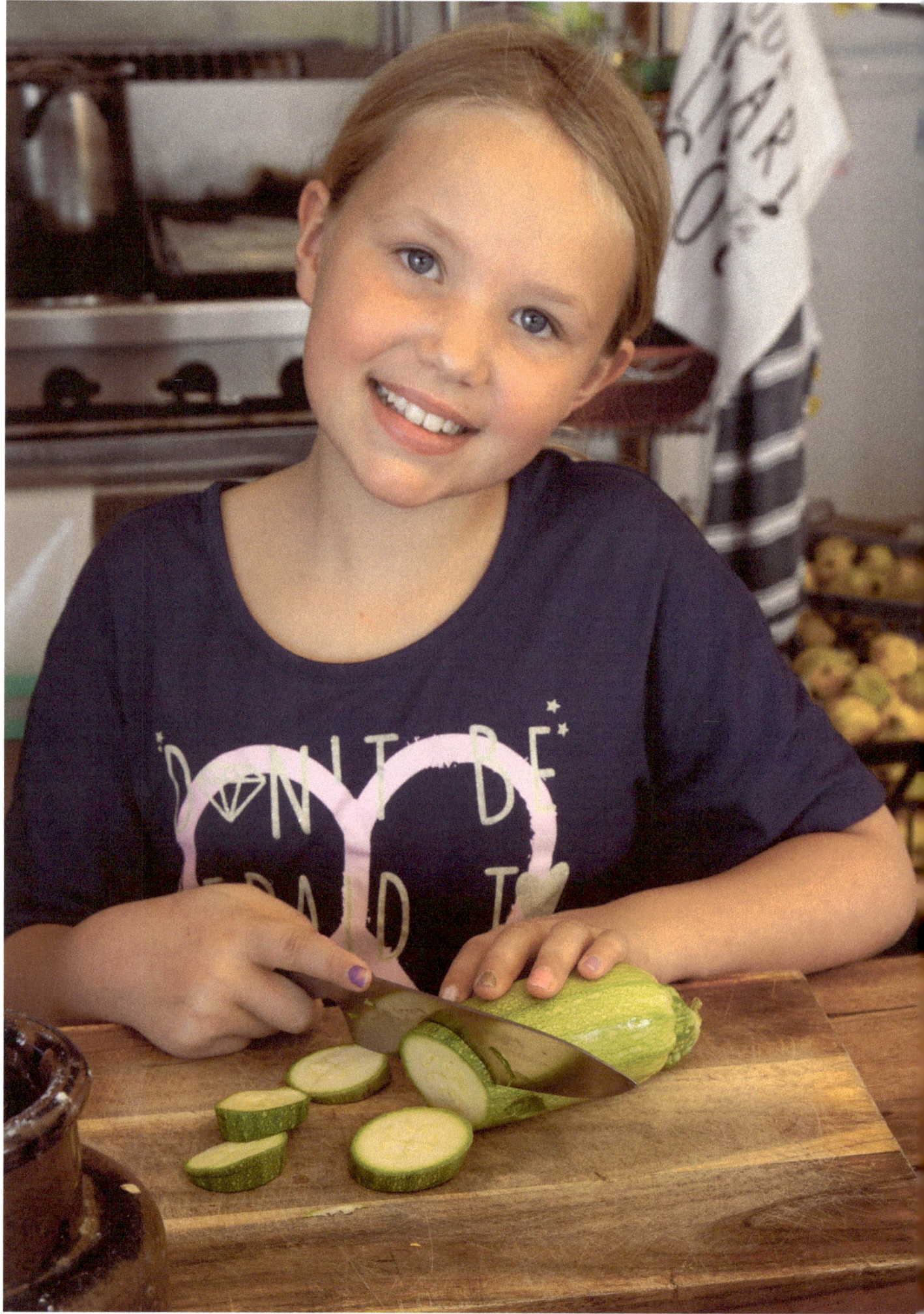

The book is divided into 8 chapters:

FROM THE PADDOCK 10

This chapter includes beef, lamb, goat and venison recipes. In Tasmania we are lucky enough to be able to be able to meet our farmers directly at the farm gate or through one of our farmers markets. Ordering your meat in bulk is generally a more economical way to purchase your meat and using all the cuts of a side adds a bit of interest to meal planning and leads to trying new recipes.

FROM THE PATCH 40

Tasmania's fertile soils provide excellent conditions to grow all sorts of fruits and vegetables at a commercial scale for a lot of the year. Picking your own berries in the summer months at fruit farms is always a popular and fun activity. Kids just love seeing what it can be turned into - it makes that jar of jam extra special. Tomatoes in season are amazing and if you preserve nothing else all year, a few jars of relish or chutney is a must in Tasmania.

WILD CAUGHT SEAFOOD 68

Commercial fishing is large industry in Tasmania, and it's especially important in regional areas. Tasmania's reputation for being a world-class seafood provider is still growing and although some species have turned into big business, there are still affordable entry-level fishing licenses available for species such as banded morwong or octopus.

FROM THE ORCHARD 88

Carts with bags of apples for a few dollars a kilo pop up all over Tasmania in autumn. It is worth a drive in the Tasmanian countryside just to buy them. Stock up on the fresh cherry seconds from the farm gate and bottle them for use through the year on dessert.

FEATHERED 108

Quail and chicken are farmed commercially and you can occasionally find a duck on a small farm.

FROM THE DAIRY 124

Tasmanian has a long history with dairy farming and cheese production. Small scale boutique cheese factories are popping up all over the island and Tasmania is becoming renowned for the cheese it produces in the state.

FROM THE SEA FARM 140

Oysters, mussels, salmon, abalone and other fish species are farmed in the pristine waters of Tasmania to the worlds best-practice standards. We are so lucky to have a reliable and safe supply of seafood all year.

FROM THE WILD 166

Wallaby, rabbit and possum are pests that are destructive to farming crops they are an excellent source of protein.

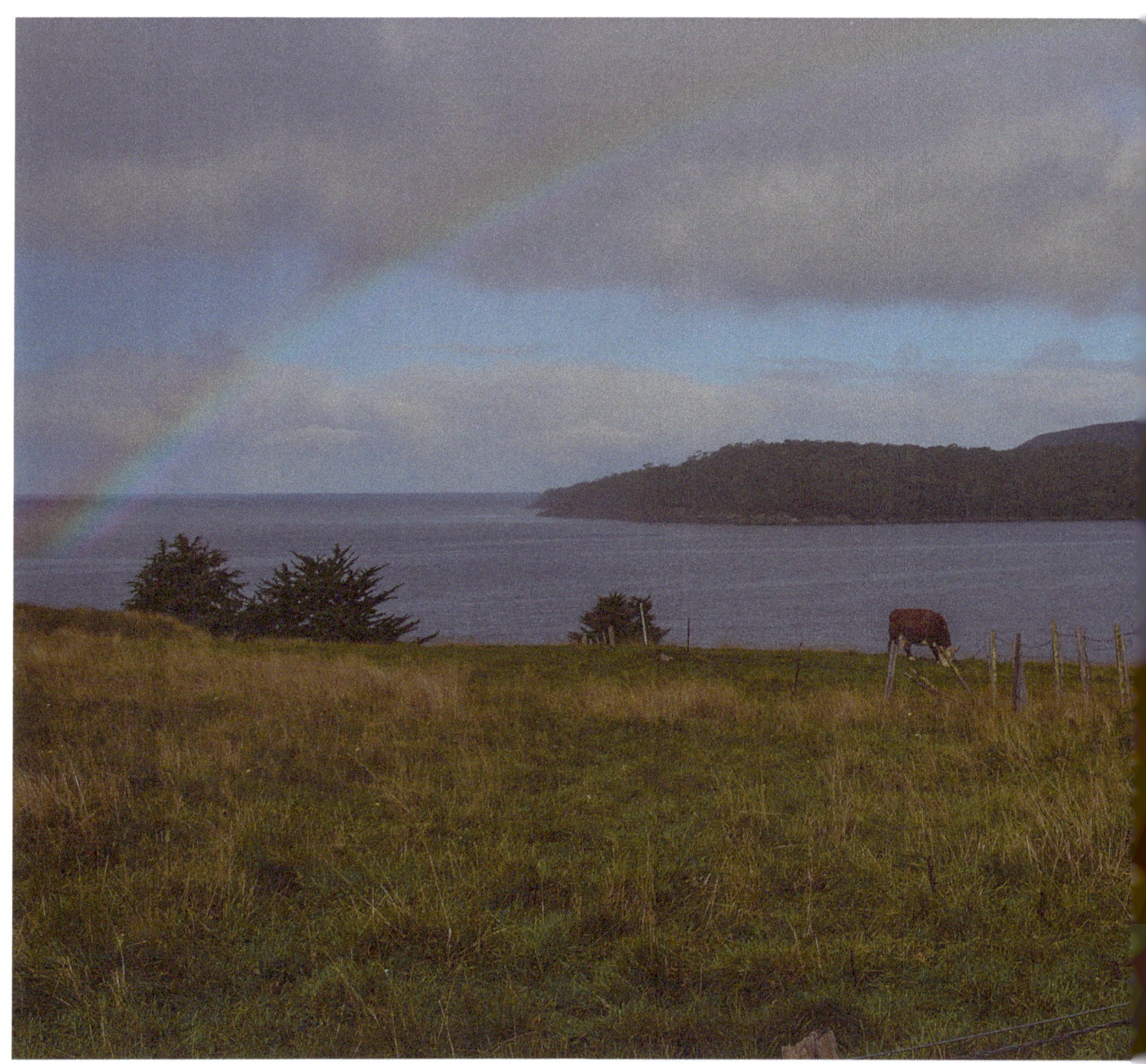

From the Paddock

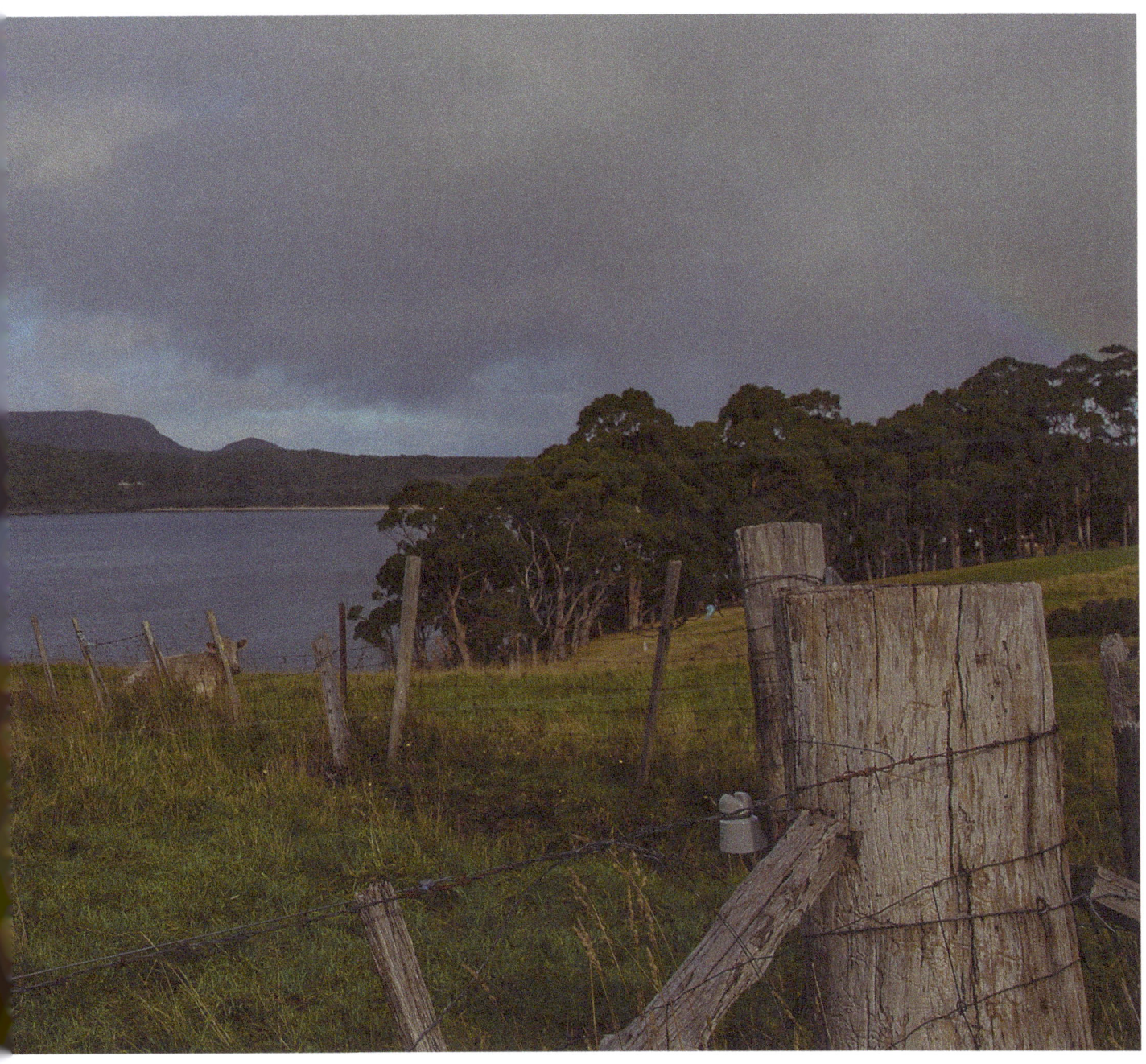

Double Cooked King Island Beef in Tasmanian Stout with Duchess Potatoes and Gremolata

SERVES 8, GENEROUSLY

Ana uses chuck for this recipe, however you can use any other cut of beef that is rich in collagen, such as the cheeks, chuck tender or oyster blade. The quantity of cream required in the mash depends on the potato variety – you may need a little more or less. This dish is delicious served with spinach that has been lightly sautéed in extra virgin olive oil and garlic. You will need to begin this recipe the day before.

DOUBLE COOKED BEEF

2 large onions

4 celery sticks

4 carrots

half chuck of beef (approximately 2.5 kilograms)

3 tablespoons extra virgin olive oil

bay leaves

20 black peppercorns

2 litres beef stock

100ml honey

2 bottles of Tasmanian stout

extra virgin olive oil

butter

DUCHESS POTATOES

1 kilogram potatoes

2 tablespoons horseradish

150ml King Island cream

salt and pepper

butter

GREMOLATA

cup chopped local parsley

zest of 1 lemon

King Island garlic cloves

To cook the beef, roughly dice the onions, celery and carrots into 2cm pieces. Remove the beef from the refrigerator, bring to room temperature and cut into 2 long pieces. Heat the oil in a large, heavy-based saucepan over medium heat, add the onions, celery, carrots, bay leaves and peppercorns, and sauté for 5 minutes, or until the vegetables start to colour. Remove the vegetables from the pan and seal the beef on all sides. Remove from the pan.

Preheat the oven to 150°C. Tip vegetables into a very large, heavy-based saucepan (or two saucepans if you don't have a big enough one) and place the beef on top of the vegetables. Pour over the beef stock, honey and stout, cover with a lid and cook in the oven for 4 -5 hours, or until the beef is very tender. Remove from the oven and let cool to room temperature.

Remove beef from the saucepan. Tip the vegetables and cooking liquid through a colander, reserving the liquid and setting the vegetables aside. Lay a large rectangle of plastic wrap on the bench. Place the beef on top and roll the beef into a tight cylinder shape, using the plastic wrap to help you form a very tight roll. Refrigerate overnight. Mash the cooked vegetables and refrigerate.

The following day, pour the cooking liquid into a small saucepan, bring to a simmer over low heat and reduce by 3/4 - this will take around 3 hours.

Preheat the oven to 160°C. Remove the beef from the fridge, take off the plastic wrap and cut into slices around 3 - 4cm thick. Heat a little olive oil and butter in an oven proof frying pan over medium heat and brown the beef slices for one minute on each side. Transfer to the oven and cook for 10 minutes. Re-heat the reserved mashed vegetables.

To make the gremolata, roughly chop the parsley, zest the lemon and crush the garlic. Mix together well and set aside.

To make the duchess potatoes, peel and roughly dice the potatoes. Tip into a saucepan, cover with water, bring to the boil over medium heat and cook for 20 minutes or until soft. Drain well, add the horseradish, cream, salt and pepper and a knob of butter, mash and stir to combine.

Serve the beef on top of the mashed vegetables, with duchess potatoes, sprinkled with gremolata and drizzled with the reduced stock.

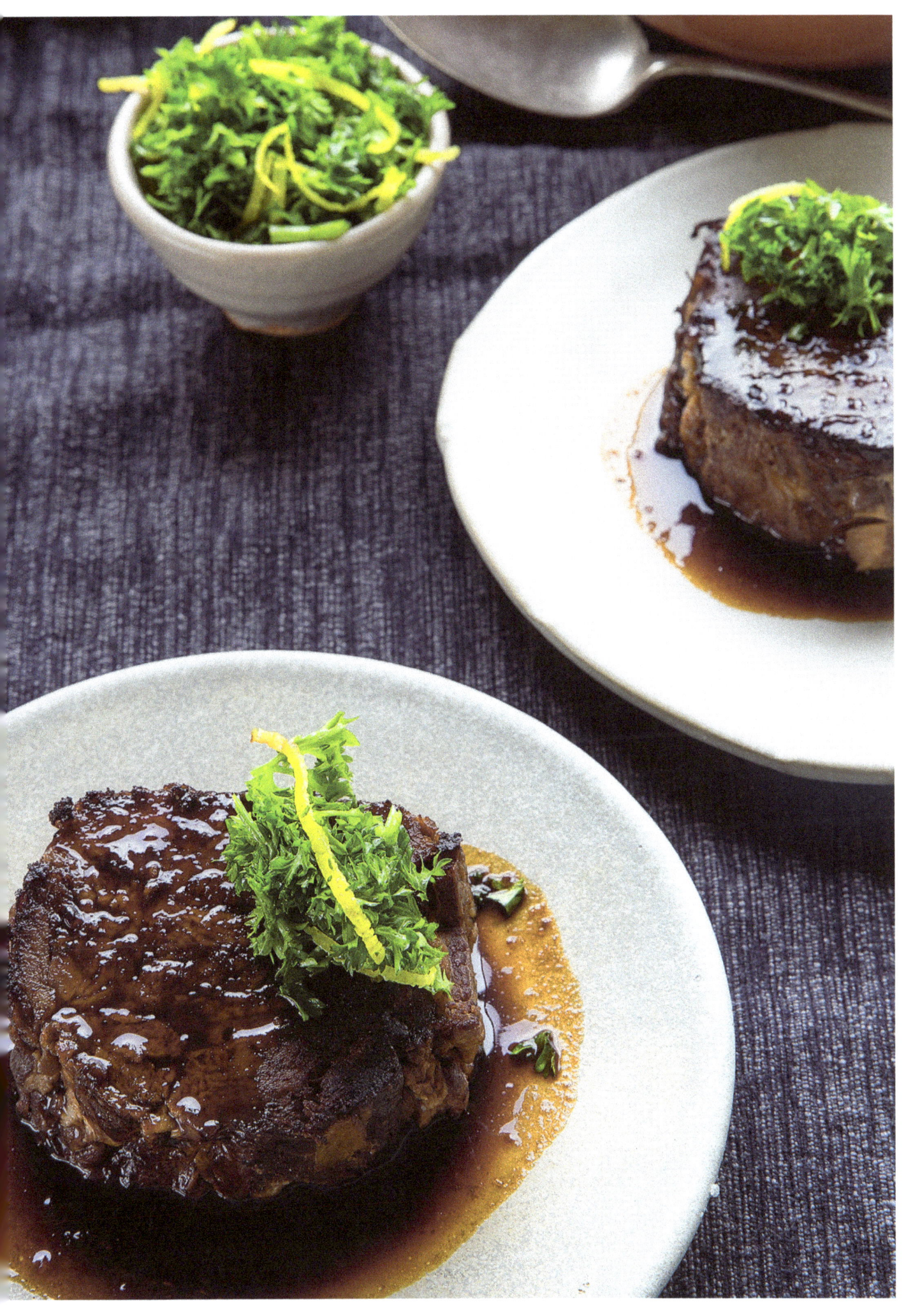

Rib Eye with a Peppercorn, Pepper Berry, Lemon and Herb Rub and Lemon Button Mushrooms

SERVES 2-4

A rib eye is a scotch fillet steak that is still on the bone - it is a big steak that can be over 600 grams in weight, so it will serve more or less people depending on how hungry everybody is feeling! This is a great meal for entertaining as much of the preparation is done ahead of time. Green peppercorns are hot, so adjust this recipe to suit your personal taste - the quantity of peppercorns here is for a mild heat. When cooking the steak, the time will vary depending on the thickness of the meat. The most accurate way to test the doneness of steak is with a meat thermometer; however resist the temptation to poke the steak repeatedly as moisture is lost with each jab. A temperature guide is: rare 45-50, medium 60-65 and well done 70-75°C. Hand cut potato chips are a wonderful accompaniment to this steak.

2 tablespoons fresh mixed herbs such as parsley, sage, rosemary

1 tablespoon green peppercorns

1 teaspoon Tasmanian pepper berries

2 beef rib eye steaks

200 grams button mushrooms

1 clove garlic

1 lemon

1 teaspoon extra virgin olive oil

1 teaspoon butter

sea salt and pepper

extra virgin olive oil for panfrying or grilling

To make the spice rub for the rib eye, roughly chop the herbs and tip into a mortar and pestle with the peppercorns and pepper berries. Pound together to form a paste. Alternatively, blend the ingredients in a food processor to make the rub. Coat the steaks on all sides with the spice rub, and marinate in the refrigerator for at least 2 hours, or preferably overnight.

To cook the beef, allow the meat to come to room temperature prior to cooking. Heat a grill, frying pan or barbecue to medium-high heat and brush the steaks with oil. Seal the steaks for 2 minutes on each side. Reduce the heat to medium and continue to cook, turning once or twice, until they are cooked to your liking. If you prefer your meat cooked above medium-rare, transfer the steaks to a baking dish and put into a hot oven to continue cooking, to avoid burning the outside. When still slightly underdone, remove the steaks from the heat, wrap in foil and rest for 10 minutes before serving.

To cook the mushrooms, wash the mushrooms and pat dry, crush the garlic and juice and zest the lemon. Heat the oil and butter in a heavy-based frying pan over low heat. Sauté the garlic for 1 minute then add the mushrooms, cook for a few minutes until well browned and soft, then add the lemon zest and juice, and season with salt and pepper.

To serve, slice up the steaks and serve with mushrooms on the side, with your choice of steamed vegetables and hand cut potato chips.

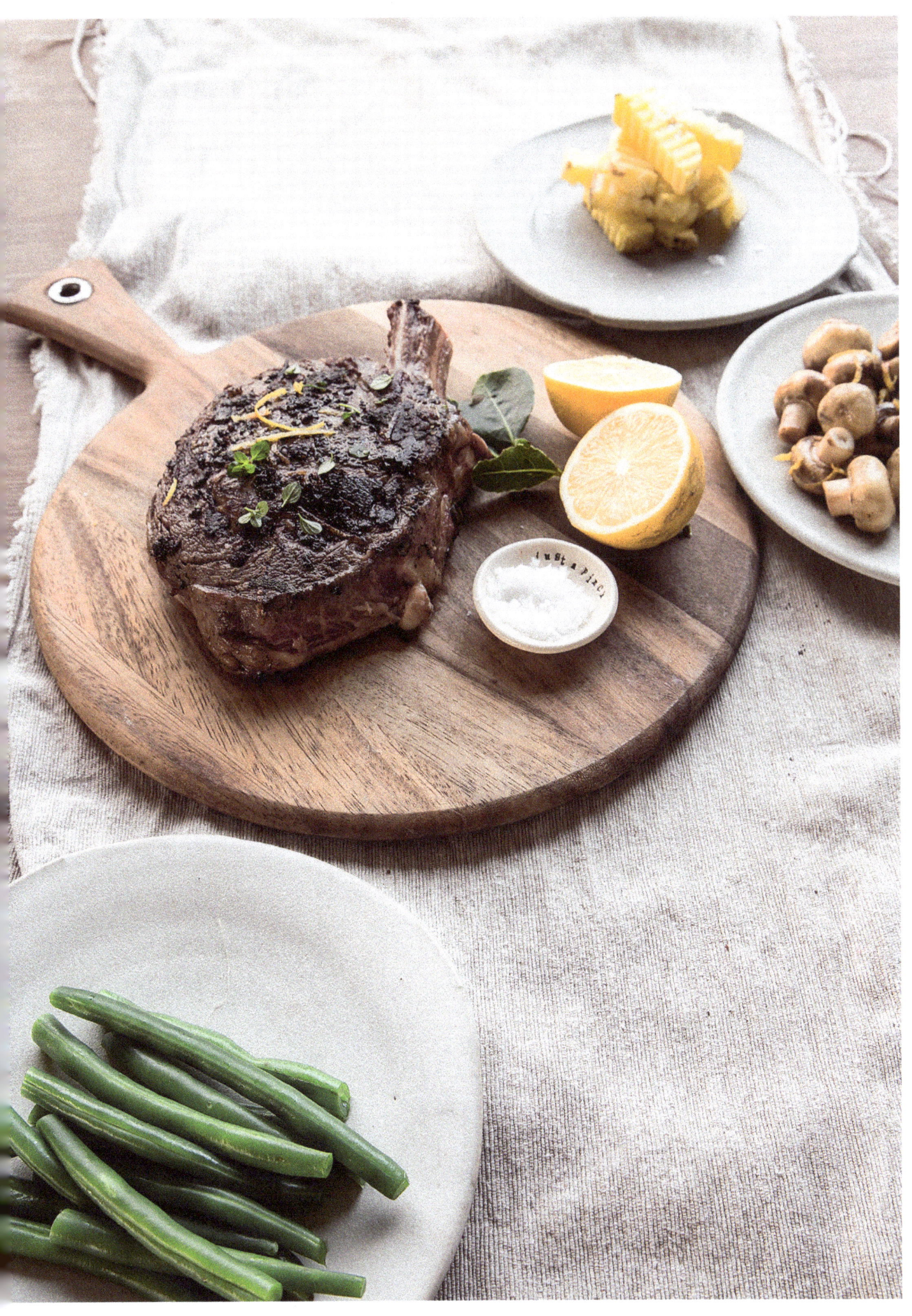

Italian Pantry Meat Balls

SERVES 8

Matt from the Italian Pantry says that this traditional recipe has been on the menu in every restaurant he has ever owned or run. It's a perfect stand-alone dish with crusty or garlic bread, with spaghetti of course, or even on a pizza. It's a dish that can be made days before a dinner party, or be in the freezer as an emergency back when friends pop in. Matt says that "this recipe is one that my grandmother taught my mother and that she passed onto me and is also lots of fun to do with kids".

TOMATO SAUCE

2 brown onions

2 cloves garlic

extra virgin olive oil

1 kilogram tomatoes

1 tablespoon basil

1 tablespoon oregano

salt and pepper

MEATBALLS

1 onion

½ clove of garlic

1 bunch flat leaf parsley

2 eggs

50 grams breadcrumbs

75 grams grated Parmesan or Pecorino Romano cheese

500 grams pork mince

500 grams beef or veal mince

4 tablespoons of tomato paste

salt and pepper to taste

1 tablespoon of Sicilian oregano

½ cup of extra virgin olive oil

To make the tomato sauce, peel and dice the onion, and crush the garlic. Tip into a heavy-based pan with a tablespoon of olive oil and sauté over low heat for 3 minutes, or until softened. Roughly chop the tomatoes, finely chop the herbs and add to the pan, bring to a simmer, cook for 25 minutes and season with salt and pepper to taste.

To make the meatballs, finely dice the onion and garlic (so small that a child will never detect them!). Finely chop or tear the parsley, depending on how rustic you would like the meatballs to appear. Using a large mixing bowl, combine the onion, garlic, parsley, eggs, breadcrumbs, cheese, minced meat, tomato paste, salt & pepper and oregano and mix well until you have the desired consistency.

Preheat the oven to 200°C. To roll the meatballs, make a well in the middle of the mix and pour in the olive oil. Roll the mix into meatballs, using the well of oil to bathe your hands as you go, to prevent sticking.

Place the meatballs in a baking dish and cook in the oven for 25-30 minutes or until they look cooked on the outside. Pour the sauce over the meatballs, reduce the temperature to 180°C and continue cooking for 40 minutes. Serve with your choice of spaghetti, crusty bread or use as a pizza topping.

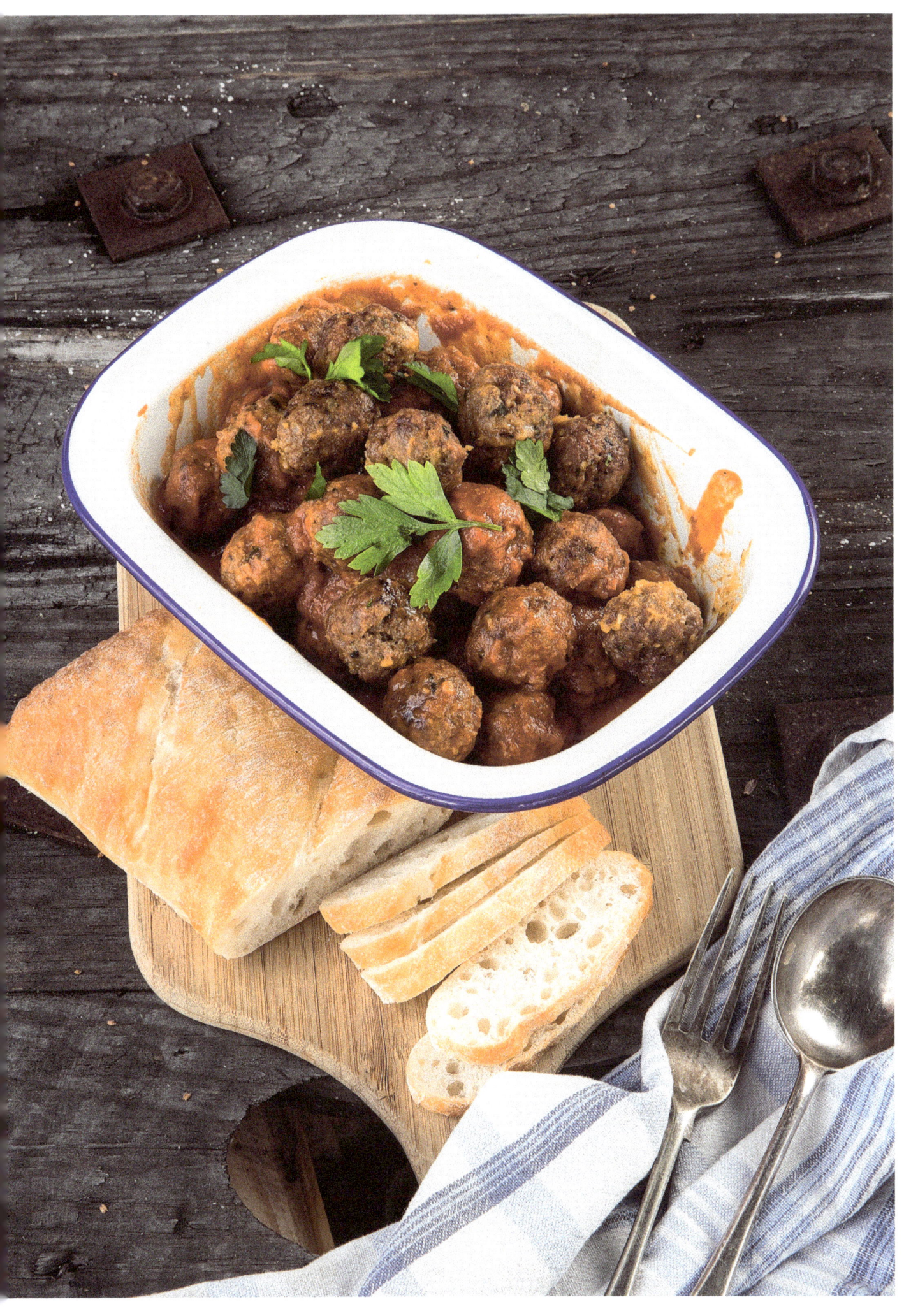

Slow Braised Lamb Shanks in Bruny Island Pinot Noir

SERVES 4

4 large lamb shanks

salt and pepper

50ml extra virgin olive oil

1 large onion

4 ripe tomatoes

1 bulb garlic

1 large sprig of thyme

400ml Bruny Island Premium Wine Pinot Noir

50 grams sugar

600ml beef stock

50 grams butter

1 bunch Italian parsley

Season the lamb shanks well with plenty of salt and pepper. Heat the oil in a large, heavy-based saucepan over medium heat and sear the lamb shanks until well browned on all sides and remove from the saucepan. Dice the onion and tomatoes and cut the bulb of garlic in half. Add the onion to the pan and cook, without colouring, for 3 minutes or until softened. Add the tomatoes, garlic and thyme and cook for 5 minutes. Add the wine and sugar, bring to the boil, reduce the heat and simmer until the liquid has reduced by half. Add the stock and then lower in the lamb shanks, bring to a simmer and cook for 2 hours, or until the meat is very tender.

When cooked, remove the lamb shanks from the sauce and set aside. Strain the sauce through a fine sieve, return to the saucepan and return to the boil. Skim off any fat, season with pepper and add a knob of butter. Return the lamb shanks to the sauce, roughly chop the parsley and sprinkle over the lamb.

Serve the lamb shanks with buttery mashed potato and seasonal greens.

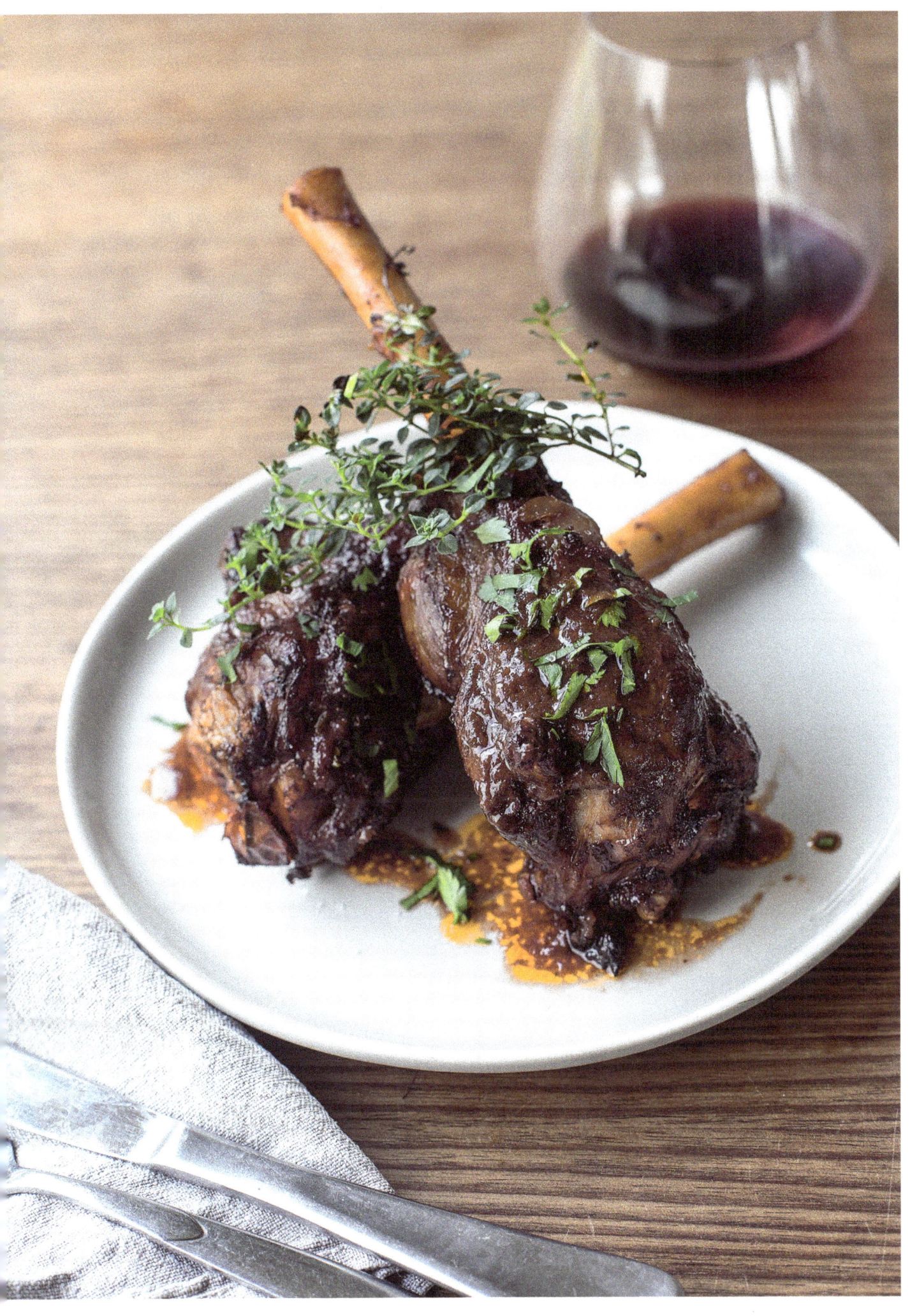

VANESSA DUNBABIN - BANGOR FARM

Hazelnut and Rosemary Crusted Bangor Lamb Racks with Pinot Noir Butter Glaze

SERVES 4

Serve these lamb racks with vegetables of your choice. You could add some baby carrots, shallots and baby beetroot to the roasting pan along with the lamb racks, and then serve with steamed green beans. For this recipe, you will need to use a baking dish that can be used in the oven as well as the stovetop.

LAMB

4 slices bread

2 cloves garlic

2 sprigs rosemary

50 grams butter

50 grams hazelnuts

salt and pepper

4 x four point lamb racks

GLAZE

2 tablespoons cold butter

500ml Bangor Pinot Noir

100ml beef stock

salt and pepper

Preheat the oven to 180°C.

Use a food processor to prepare the crust. Add the bread to the processor and process into crumbs, remove and set aside. Peel the garlic cloves and remove the rosemary leaves from the woody stems. Add the garlic, rosemary leaves, butter, hazelnuts and a good pinch of sea salt and cracked pepper, and process until smooth. Add the breadcrumbs and combine well. Remove any visible fat and sinew from the lamb rack and press the crust firmly onto the meaty side of the rack. The crust should be approximately 1/2 cm thick.

Carefully place the lamb racks into a baking dish, crust side down (additional vegetables of your choice can also be added the baking dish at this point). Bake in the oven for 10 minutes.

Remove from the oven and carefully turn the lamb racks so that the crust side is facing up. Return to the oven and continue to cook until the lamb is done to your liking. The lamb racks will require a total cooking time of approximately 25 minutes to be cooked to medium – adjust the cooking time if required so that the lamb is cooked to your liking. Remove from the oven, wrap the lamb racks in foil and set aside to rest. Return the vegetables to the oven to finish cooking if required, then remove and keep warm while you make the glaze.

To make the glaze, place the baking pan on the stovetop over low heat. Cut the butter into small cubes. Pour the wine and stock into the pan, season with salt and pepper, and stir with a wooden spoon to loosen any remnants on the bottom of the pan. Simmer the glaze until 1/3 of the liquid has reduced, and then remove from the heat. Whilst the pan is still hot, quickly whisk the butter into the glaze. If the butter doesn't quite melt, return briefly to the heat, but take care not to overheat, otherwise the glaze will split.

To serve, pour the glaze over the lamb racks and vegetables and enjoy with a glass of Bangor Pinot Noir.

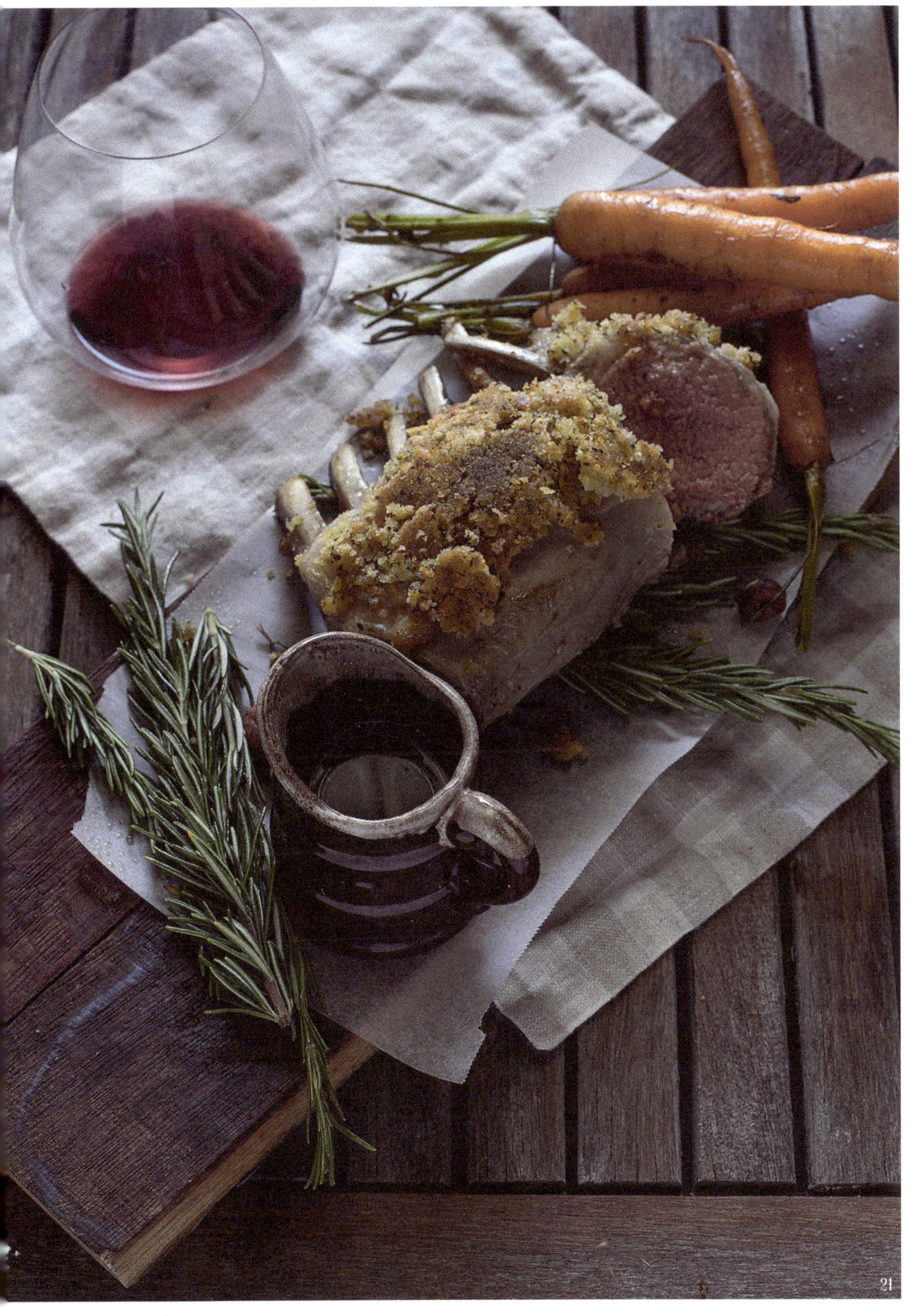

KATE FIELD - LEAP FARM

Beef, Mushroom and Red Wine Pie

SERVES 4

This hearty, homemade pie has gorgeously rich gravy and tender chunks of meat. To make the pie gluten free, substitute a gluten free pastry and skip dusting the beef with flour before browning. This pie tastes even better if you make your own beef stock and use a really good red wine in the filling, and you could also make your own shortcrust pastry if you have time! Kate from Leap Farm suggests that if you just can't wait for the mixture to cool before baking it into a pie – simply serve with mash and peas instead, it's absolutely delicious.

900 grams Leap Farm round beef steak

plain flour for dusting

50 grams butter

extra virgin olive oil

1 small brown onion

2 cloves of garlic

4-5 large mushrooms

dried thyme to taste

salt and pepper

1 beef stock cube, crumbled

1 glass of good red wine

3 tomatoes

2 sheets puff pastry

1 egg yolk

To make the pie filling, roughly chop the round steak into 2-3cm cubes. Dust the cubes in plain flour (to do this, add the flour to a small zip-lock bag, then add the steak in two batches - jiggle it around and then after it's all dusted, you can just throw the bag into the rubbish). Heat a large, heavy-based saucepan over medium heat, add the butter and a good splash of oil. Add half of the beef to the pan and cook, turning until well browned on all sides. Finely dice the onion, and add to the saucepan with the remaining beef. Crush the garlic and add to the pan along with the first lot of beef, and add a little more olive oil if the mixture is starting to stick. Roughly chop the mushrooms and add to the saucepan with the thyme, one teaspoon of black pepper, the stock cube, wine and a splash of water. Roughly dice the tomatoes and add to the saucepan. Stirring gently, bring the mixture to the boil and reduce to a simmer – a rich, dark gravy should be developing. Continue to simmer for 20 minutes, taste and season to taste. Reduce heat to low and continue to simmer for 1-2 hours until the meat is very tender. Set aside to cool.

To create the pie, pre heat the oven to 180°C. Line a 20cm round pie tin with puff pastry. Pour the cooled pie mixture into the tin, leaving approximately 1cm of space at the top of the dish. Cut a circle of pastry to fit the top and seal the edges by pressing the layers of pastry together with a fork. Whisk the egg yolk, and use to brush the top of the pie. Bake in the oven for 25 - 35 minutes, or until the pastry is golden brown and the pie filling is piping hot – you should be able to see some bubbling at the edge of the pastry lid.

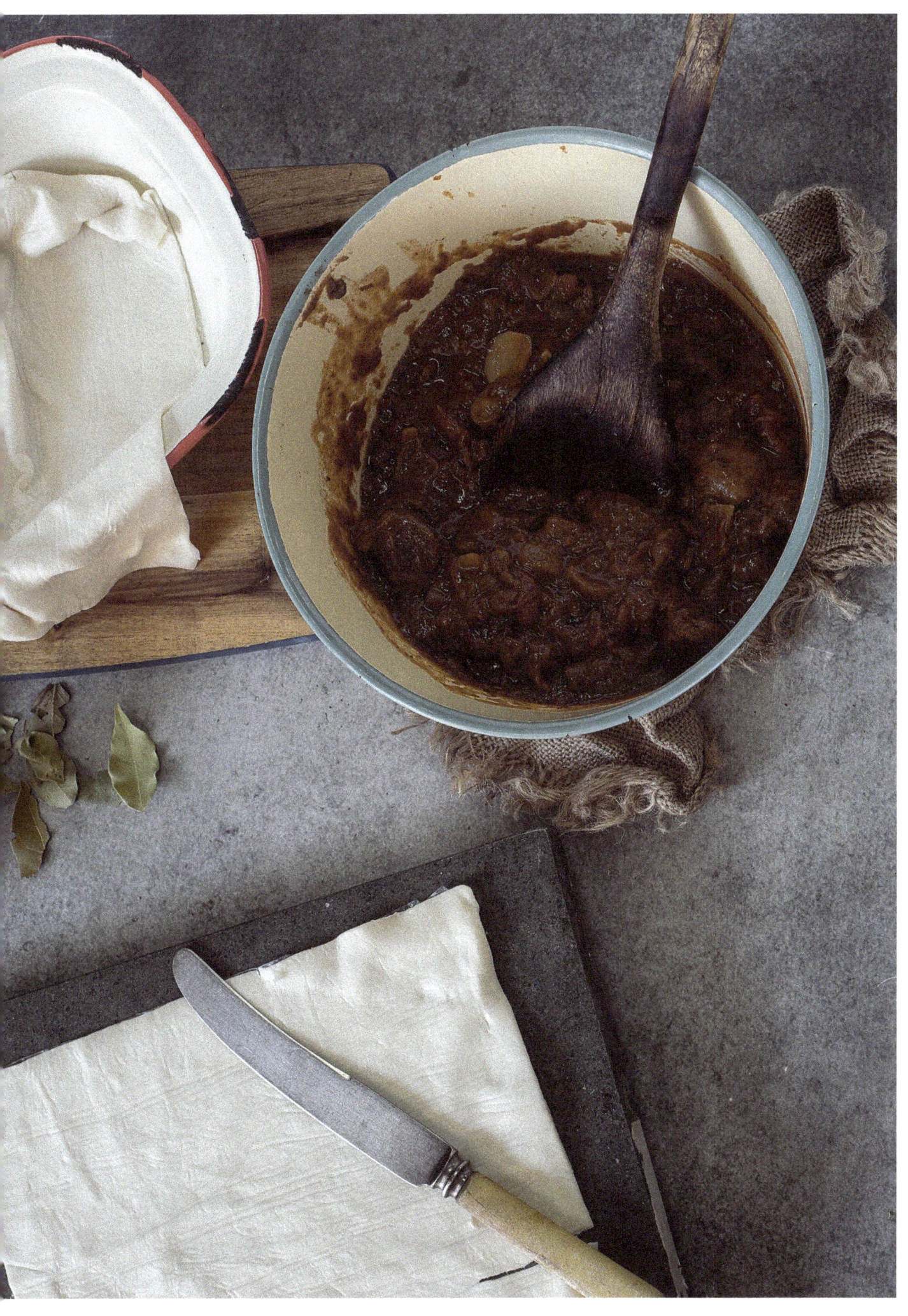

Normandy Pork in Spreyton Fresh Cider with Apples, Celery and Walnuts

SERVES 4

Fresh and fruity, this pork casserole with celery and walnuts comes from Normandy in northwestern France, where cider apples grow in profusion. Traditionally, a dish of rice is cooked in the oven at the same time, making this a very simple meal to prepare. Try using an apple variety such as Jonathan or Royal Gala and serve the finished dish with green vegetables.

500 gram pork fillet

8 celery stalks

1 onion

2 tablespoons extra virgin olive oil

1 ¾ cups Spreyton Fresh cider (Classic or Vintage Cider)

1 bay leaf

black pepper

4 cups chicken stock

1 ½ cups long grain rice

3 red-skinned apples

¾ cup crushed walnuts

Preheat the oven to 160°C.

Trim the pork fillet of visible fat and cut into 2-3cm cubes. Remove the celery leaves from the stalks, cut stalks into 5 cm lengths and roughly chop the leaves. Roughly chop the onion and set aside. Heat the oil in a flameproof casserole dish, add the diced pork and fry, stirring frequently, for 5 minutes or until browned on all sides. Add the celery stalks and the onion and fry gently for about 10 minutes or until softened. Pour in the Spreyton Fresh Cider, add the bay leaf and season with pepper to taste. Bring to a boil, then cover the dish and transfer to the oven. Cook for 1 ¼ hours, or until the pork is tender.

Approximately 40 minutes before the end of the cooking time, bring the stock to the boil and pour the rice into an ovenproof dish. Pour over the hot stock, stir well, cover and put in the oven to cook with the pork.

Approximately 25 minutes before the end of the cooking time, quarter and core the apples but do not peel. Thickly slice the quarters, then add to the pork, cover and return the dish to the oven to finish cooking.

Meanwhile, toast the walnuts by heating a small frying pan over medium heat. Add the walnuts and cook, stirring, until lightly toasted.

After 1 ¼ hours, remove the pork from the oven and check that the meat is tender. Stir in the toasted walnuts and taste for pepper. To serve, garnish the pork with the reserved chopped celery leaves and serve hot, accompanied by the rice.

VARIATIONS:

Add 1 clove of chopped garlic and 1 teaspoon chopped fresh ginger to the dish along with the onion, and use freshly squeezed orange juice in place of the cider.

Replace the apple slices with the segments of 2 oranges, adding them 10 minutes before the end of the cooking time. Garnish the casserole with shreds of orange rind. Cook the rice in a mixture of orange juice and vegetable stock.

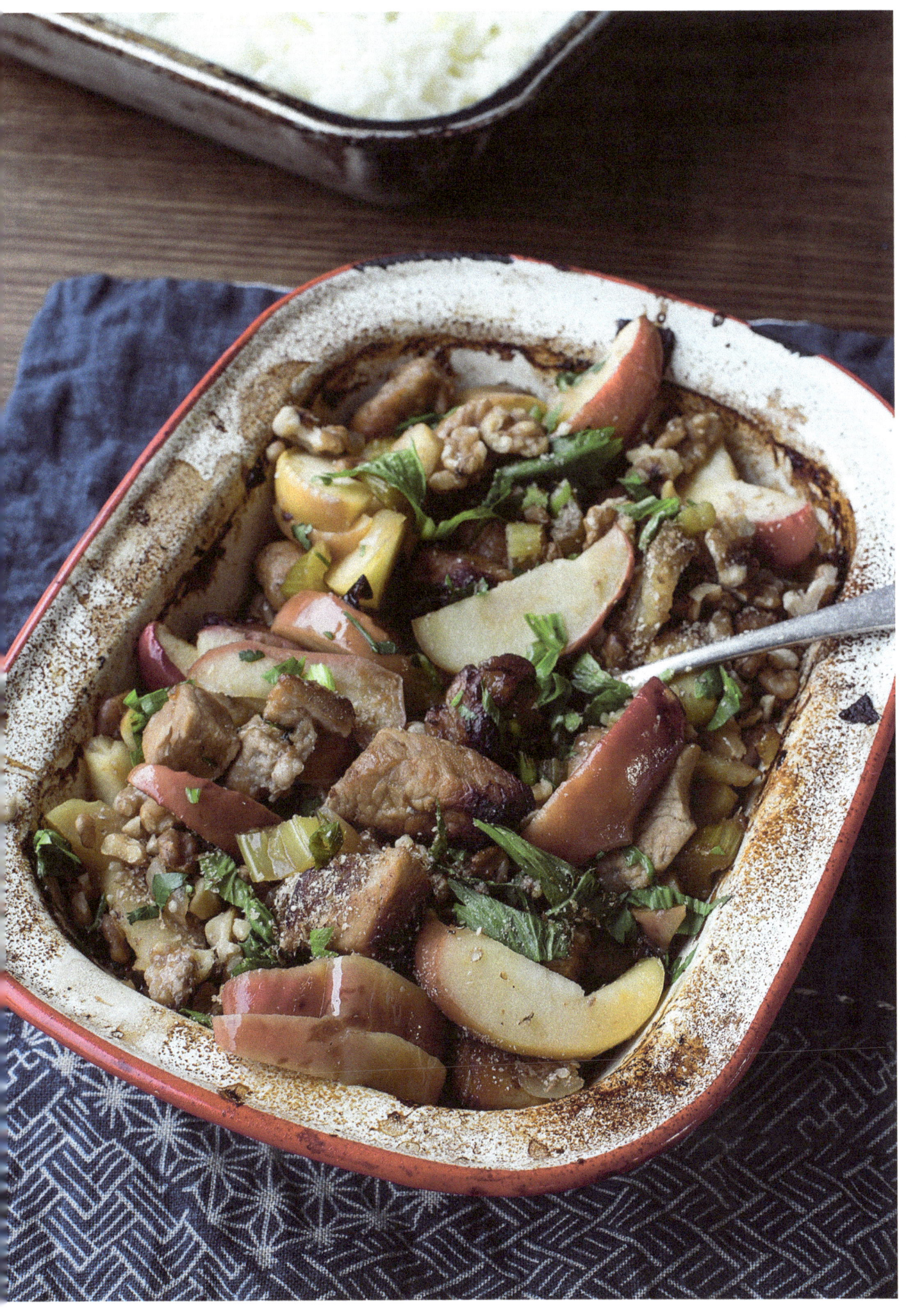

Thai Venison Salad

SERVES 4

The venison gives this traditional Thai salad a delicious gamey flavour that pairs so well with the punchy flavours in the dressing. Substitute eye fillet of beef if venison is not available and serve with rice noodles for a more substantial dish.

SALAD

500 grams venison backstrap

2 cloves garlic

3 tablespoons light soy sauce

2 tablespoons lime juice

1 cucumber

3 spring onions

⅓ cup mint leaves

⅓ cup Thai basil leaves

⅓ cup coriander

200 grams mesculun salad mix

DRESSING

2 long red chillies

3 tablespoons light soy sauce

2 tablespoons lime juice

2 teaspoons palm sugar

2 kaffir lime leaves

To marinate the venison, crush the garlic and mix with the soy sauce and lime juice. Pour over the venison fillet and marinate for 10 minutes.

To cook the venison, heat the barbecue, grill or a heavy-based frying pan over high heat and sear the venison on all sides, cooking for 3-5 minutes on each side, depending on thickness – this timing will cook the meat to rare, so adjust the cooking time to your preference. Remove the pan from the heat, cover the venison with foil and allow to rest for 5 minutes.

To make the salad, slice the cucumber and spring onions and finely chop the herbs. Mix the cucumber, mesculun, spring onions and herbs together and arrange on a large serving platter.

To make the dressing, finely slice the chillies, finely slice the lime leaves, grate the palm sugar and combine all dressing ingredients, stirring until the palm sugar has dissolved.

To serve, slice the venison into thin slices, arrange on top of the salad and drizzle with the dressing.

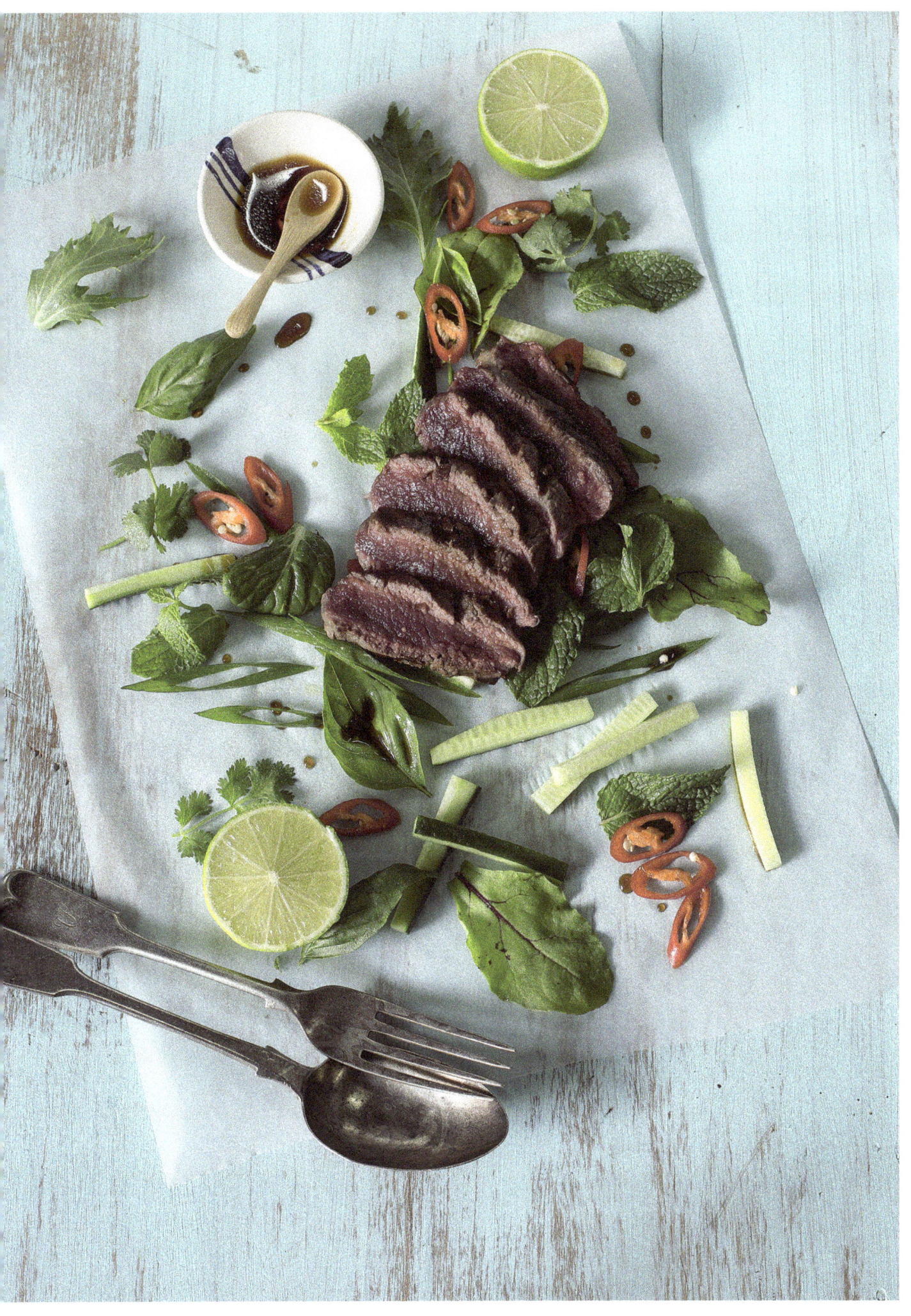

KATE FIELD - LEAP FARM

Moroccan Inspired Goat Kebabs

SERVES 4-6

These kebabs are made in a traditional style, using goat mince rather than chunks of meat. To shape the meat around the skewer, wet your hands slightly and scoop up a handful of mince. Shape the meat around the skewer, turning as you go to form a 'sausage' shape. You could also form the mixture into balls to serve as a canapé or at a party with a bowl of tzatziki alongside. Ras al Hanout is a Moroccan spice created from a mixture of spices – the recipe for making your own is below.

1 brown onion

4 tablespoons mint leaves

500 grams minced Leap Farm goat meat

1 teaspoon of freshly ground black pepper

1 teaspoon of salt

1 teaspoon of Ras al Hanout (optional)

Bamboo skewers

Grate the onion and finely chop the mint. Mix all of the ingredients together in a large bowl, then cover and place in the refrigerator to chill for one hour. While the mixture is chilling, soak the bamboo skewers in cold water.

Form the kebabs by moulding the mince mix around the skewers, into a sausage shape. Brush each kebab lightly with olive oil.

To cook the skewers, heat the barbecue, grill or a heavy-based pan over medium heat. Cook the skewers for 10 -15 minutes, turning every 3 minutes, or until cooked through and well browned. Serve with tzatziki and salad.

RAS AL HANOUT
MAKES APPROXIMATELY 50 GRAMS

1 teaspoon of cumin seeds

1 teaspoon of coriander seeds

6 cardamom pods, seeds only

½ teaspoon fennel seeds

½ teaspoon of black peppercorns

2 teaspoons sweet paprika

1 teaspoon of cinnamon powder

1 teaspoon turmeric

1 teaspoon cayenne pepper

1 teaspoon salt

½ teaspoon allspice

½ teaspoon sugar

To toast the spices, heat a small frying pan over medium heat and add the cumin, coriander, cardamom, fennel and peppercorns. Stir continuously for a couple of minutes, or until lightly toasted and fragrant. Tip into a mortar and pestle (or a spice grinder) and grind into a powder – use a fine sieve to remove the husks if you wish. Mix together with the remaining ingredients, tip into a zip-lock bag or jar and store in the freezer to keep fresh.

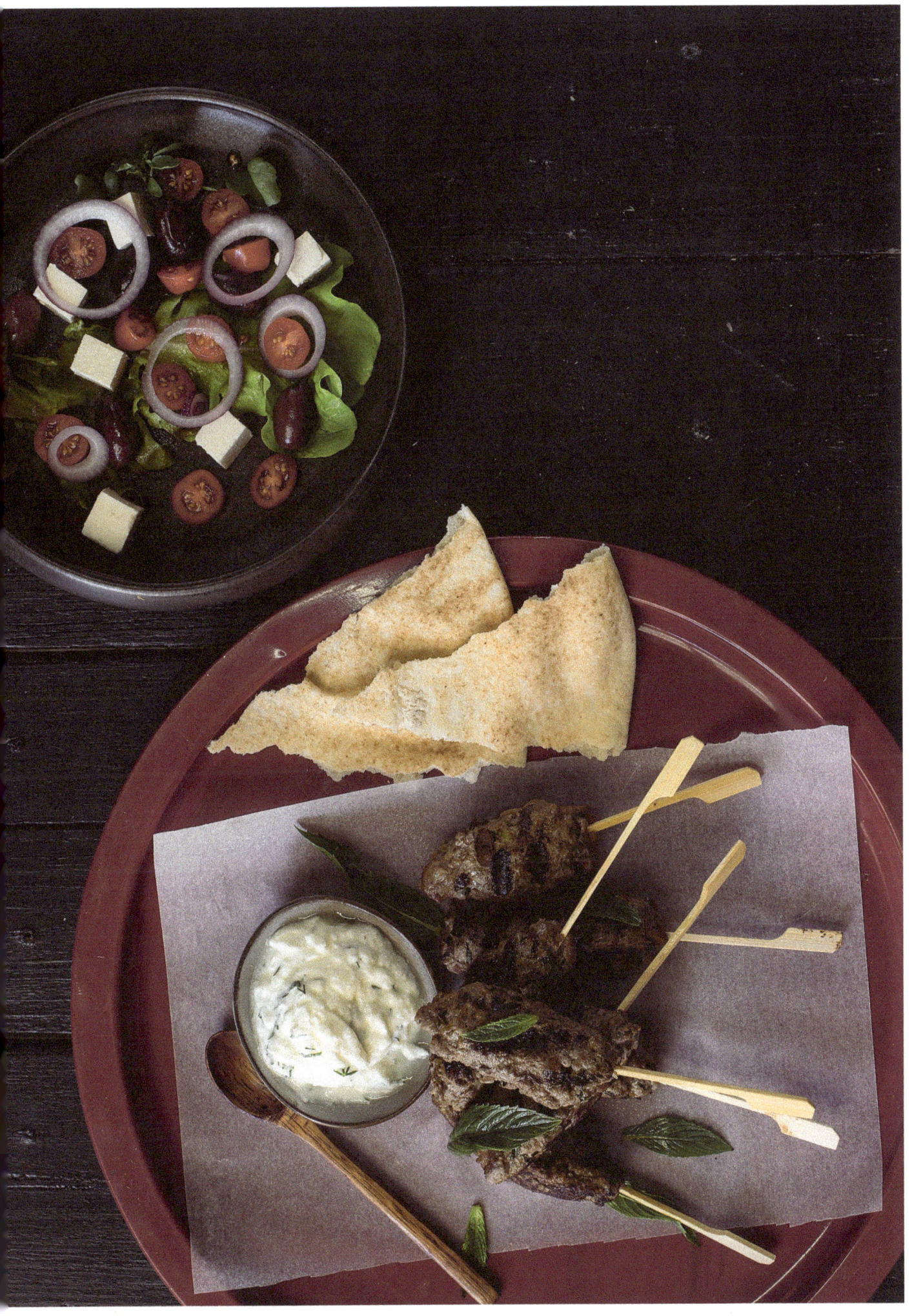

Slow Cooked Leap Farm Goat Shanks

SERVES 4

Pepper berries are grown in Tasmania, and they impart a deliciously hot, sweet and aromatic flavour to dishes. They can be used in both sweet and savoury dishes and, like black peppercorns, they can be ground in a pepper grinder or in a mortar and pestle. If you don't have a slow cooker, simply brown the shanks in a heavy-based casserole dish, add the remaining ingredients, cover and cook in the oven at 160°C for 2-3 hours.

4 Leap Farm goat shanks

1 tablespoon extra virgin olive oil

2 onions

2 cloves garlic

400 grams tomatoes

4 sprigs thyme

200ml beef stock

2 bay leaves

½ teaspoon pepper berries

200ml red wine

salt

Heat the oil in a large, heavy-based saucepan over medium heat. Seal the shanks on each side until browned, and transfer to the slow cooker. Peel and roughly chop the onions and garlic, chop the tomatoes and add to the slow cooker. Add the thyme, stock, bay leaves, cracked pepper berries, wine and a pinch of salt. Set the slow cooker to cook for 4 hours on high heat. The goat shanks will be soft, tender and falling away from the bone. Serve with a mixed vegetable mash, such as potato, sweet potato and pumpkin, or with polenta and vegetables.

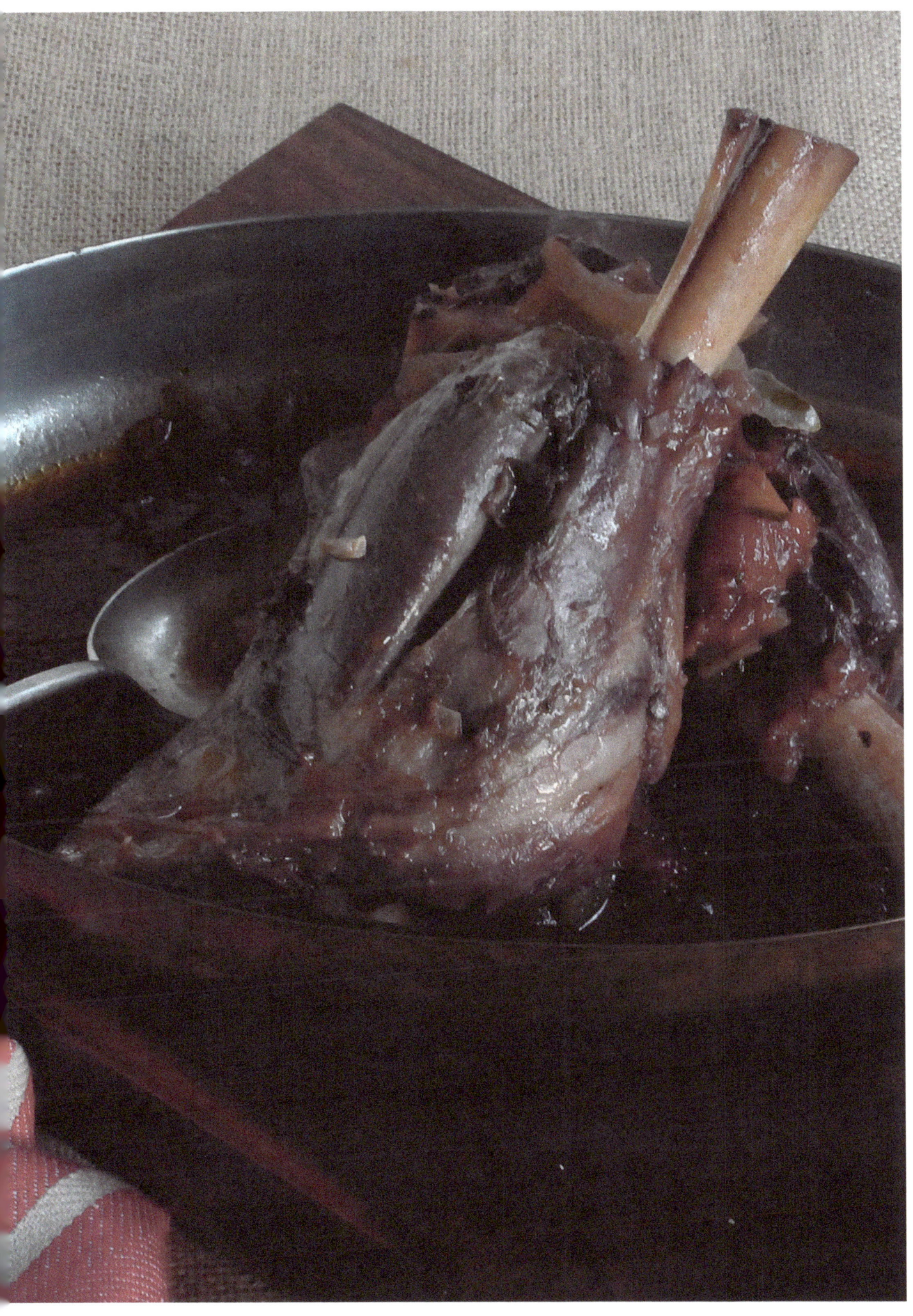

Minestrone Soup

SERVES 8

Homemade minestrone soup is hearty and heart-warming and this is such a versatile recipe. You can add any other vegetables that you like – try peas, green beans corn, or whatever is in season. This soup tastes even better with homemade stock, my recipe for beef stock can be found at eloiseemmett.com

2 onions

2 cloves garlic

2 rashers bacon

2 stalks celery

3 medium carrots

extra virgin olive oil

1 tablespoon basil

1 teaspoon oregano

400 grams tomatoes

1 litre beef stock

200 grams small pasta

400 grams cooked kidney or cannellini beans

salt and cracked pepper

Peel and finely dice the onion, crush the garlic, and finely chop the bacon, celery and carrots. Heat the oil in a large saucepan over medium heat, add the onion, garlic, bacon, celery and carrots and sauté for 3 minutes or until softened.

Add the herbs, tomatoes and stock, bring to the boil, reduce the heat and simmer for 20 minutes. Add the pasta (any other vegetables you would like to include can be also be added now) and continue to simmer until the pasta is cooked. Add the beans and season to taste with salt and pepper.

To serve, top with grated Parmesan Cheese and some homemade garlic pizza bread.

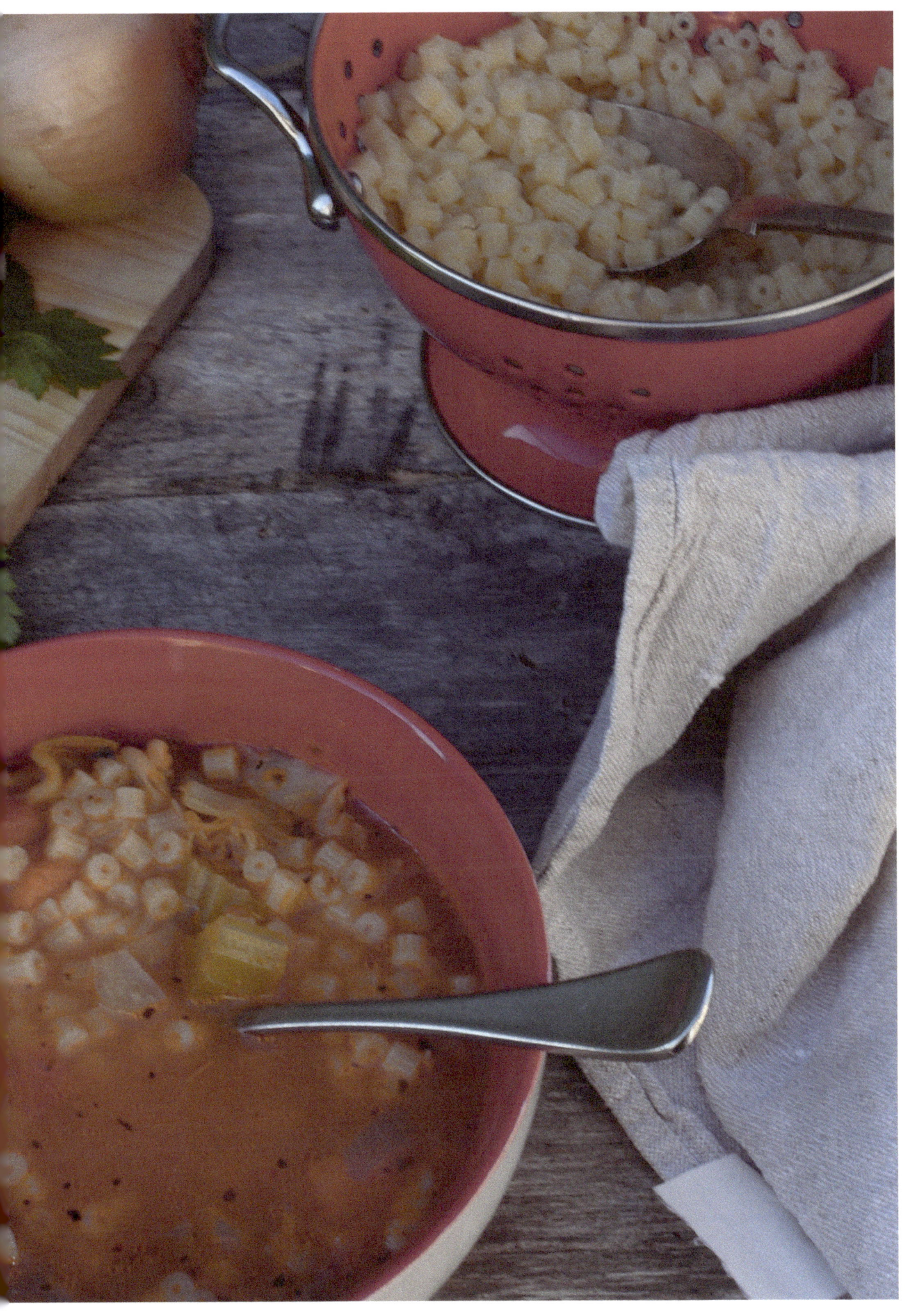

Barbecued French Toast with Bacon and Maple Syrup

SERVES 4

I love this recipe and cook it all the time – it's the perfect way to create a special breakfast for a large group and is also really easy to make as a fancy camping breakfast.

2 eggs

1 cup milk

salt and pepper

extra virgin olive oil spray, for greasing

4 rashers bacon

4 thick slices bread

1 tablespoon butter

4 tablespoons maple syrup

Using a large bowl, whisk together the egg and the milk and season with a little salt and pepper. Heat the flat grill plate of the barbecue to low heat. Spray with oil, lay the rashers of bacon on the hottest part of the grill and cook until crispy.

Meanwhile, dip each slice of bread into the egg mix, put 4 small lumps of the butter on the cooler part of the grill plate, and carefully place one piece of bread on top of each lump of butter. Cook the bread for approximately two minutes on each side, or until golden brown.

To serve, top each slice of French toast with a rasher of bacon and drizzle with maple syrup.

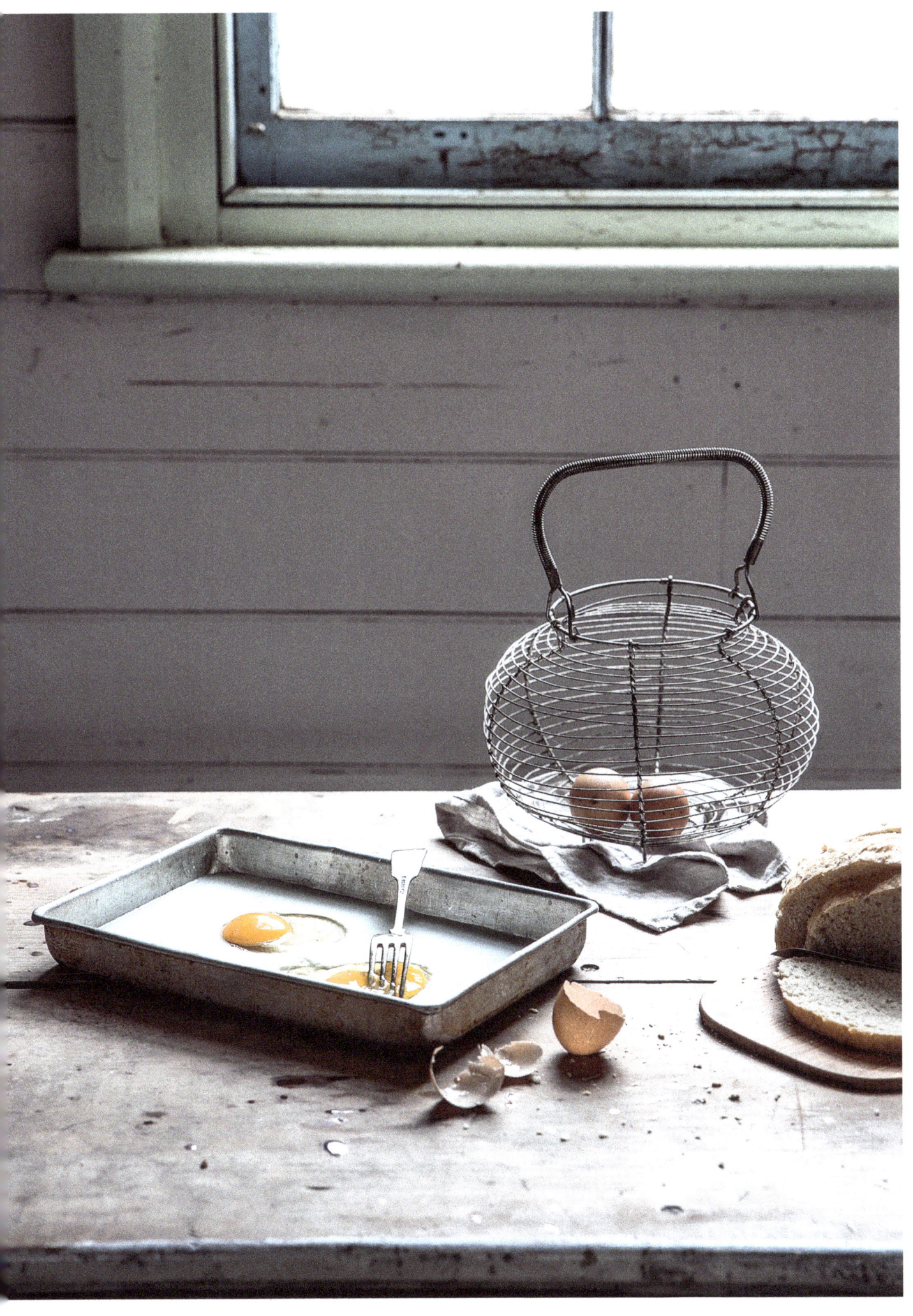

Honey and Garlic Braised Bangor Farm Lamb Shanks with Pasta and Roast Pumpkin

SERVES 4

2 Bangor Farm lamb shanks

1 tablespoon extra virgin olive oil

3 tablespoons flour

1 brown onion

3 cloves garlic

2 sprigs rosemary

2 cups tomatoes (or use a can of crushed tomatoes)

1 tablespoon honey

2 cups beef stock

salt and pepper

200 grams pumpkin

2 cups silverbeet

500 grams fettuccini pasta
see page 158 to make your own pasta

200ml cream

100 grams Parmesan cheese

Heat the oil in a large, heavy-based saucepan over medium heat. Coat the lamb shanks with flour, add to the saucepan and brown the meat on all sides. Slice the onions, crush the garlic and chop the rosemary leaves and tomatoes. Transfer the shanks to the slow cooker, and add the onions, garlic, rosemary, tomatoes, honey, stock and a pinch of salt and pepper.

Cook on high for 4 hours, or until the meat is falling off the bone. If you have time, turn off the slow cooker, cool the shanks to room temperature, then refrigerate for 2 hours to encourage the fat to settle on the surface. Remove all the fat from the top of the dish and discard all fat and bones.

Use a fork to break up the meat slightly, and tip all of the meat and sauce into a heavy-based pan. Bring to a simmer until slightly reduced and thickened.

Preheat the oven to 180°C. Dice the pumpkin into

1.5 cm cubes, tip into a roasting pan, drizzle with extra virgin olive oil and cook in the oven for 25 minutes or until cooked through and golden. Wash and shred the silver beet. Cook the pasta in salted boiling water according to packet instructions, and drain.

Add the cream to the saucepan with the meat and sauce, and continue to reduce for about 5 minutes, or until the sauce has thickened. Toss the roasted pumpkin and silverbeet through the sauce, and cook for a few minutes or until the silver beet has softened.

To serve, toss the hot pasta through the sauce and top with grated Parmesan cheese.

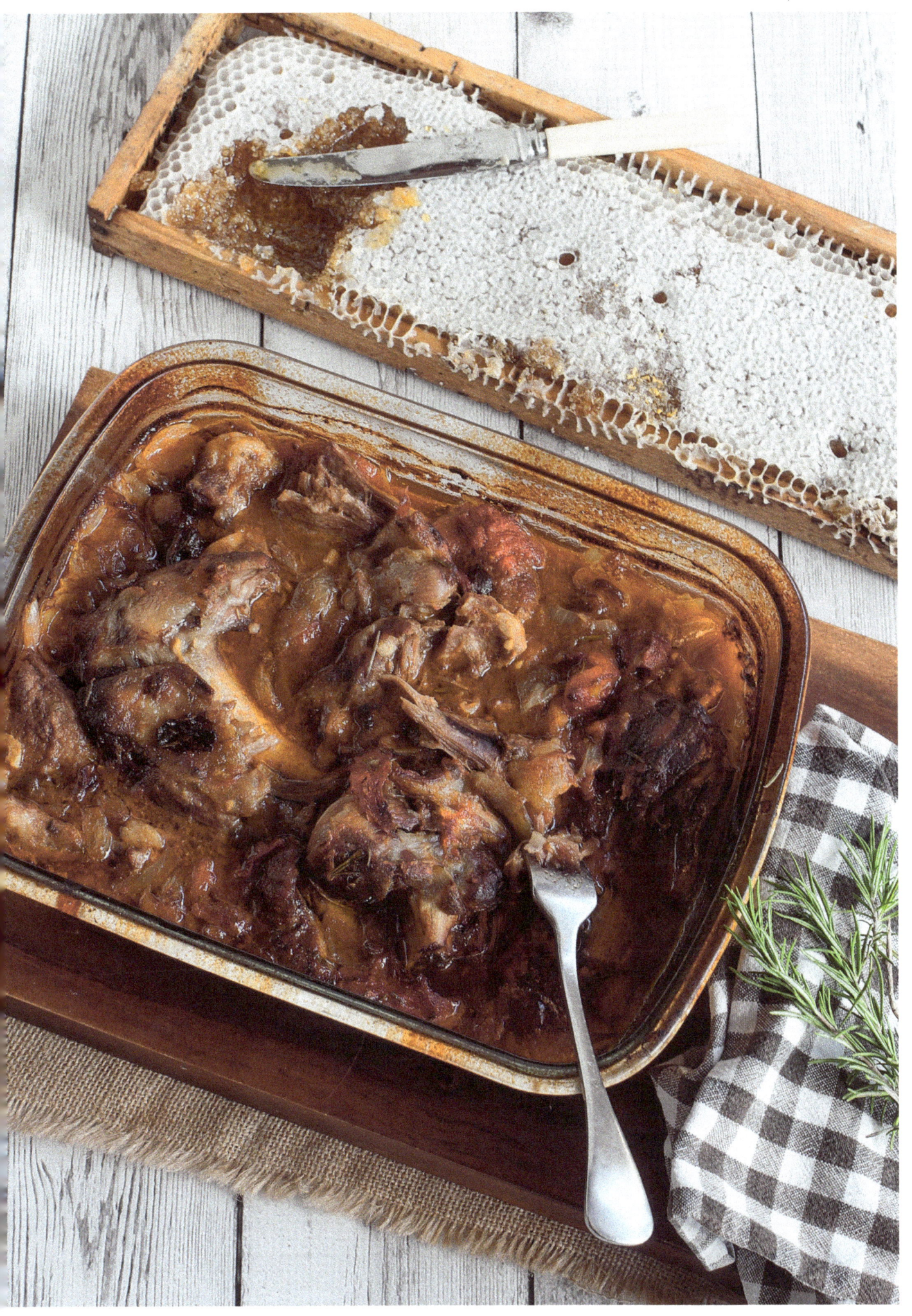

Venison Carpaccio

SERVES 4 AS A ENTRÉE OR LIGHT LUNCH

Carpaccio is a classic Italian dish, and is simple to make - as long as you can slice the venison very thinly. Traditionally, the dish is made with raw beef and truffles, and it would also be garnished with an excellent Parmesan cheese. If you prefer the venison to be cured, you can leave it to marinate in the acidic lemon juice and vinegar, and you could also experiment with different vinegars and herbs to change up the flavours.

320 grams venison fillet

1 tablespoon red wine vinegar

1 tablespoon lemon juice

2 tablespoons extra virgin olive oil

1 tablespoon capers

1 tablespoon fresh basil, dill and/or parsley

50 grams Parmesan cheese

shaved truffle or truffle oil

cracked black pepper

sea salt

Using a very shape knife, slice the venison very thinly (you should be able to see light through the slices) and arrange the thin slices on a platter, or on 4 individual plates.

Drizzle the vinegar and lemon juice over the venison. If you prefer, at this stage you can leave the venison to cure for ten minutes to one hour, or just serve it immediately (I like to serve mine straight away).

Drizzle the venison with the olive oil, finely chop the capers and herbs and sprinkle over the venison. Finally, add the thinly shaved Parmesan and the shaved truffles (or truffle oil), pepper and sea salt.

Serve with some crusty bread or grissini to mop up the delicious vinegar and oil.

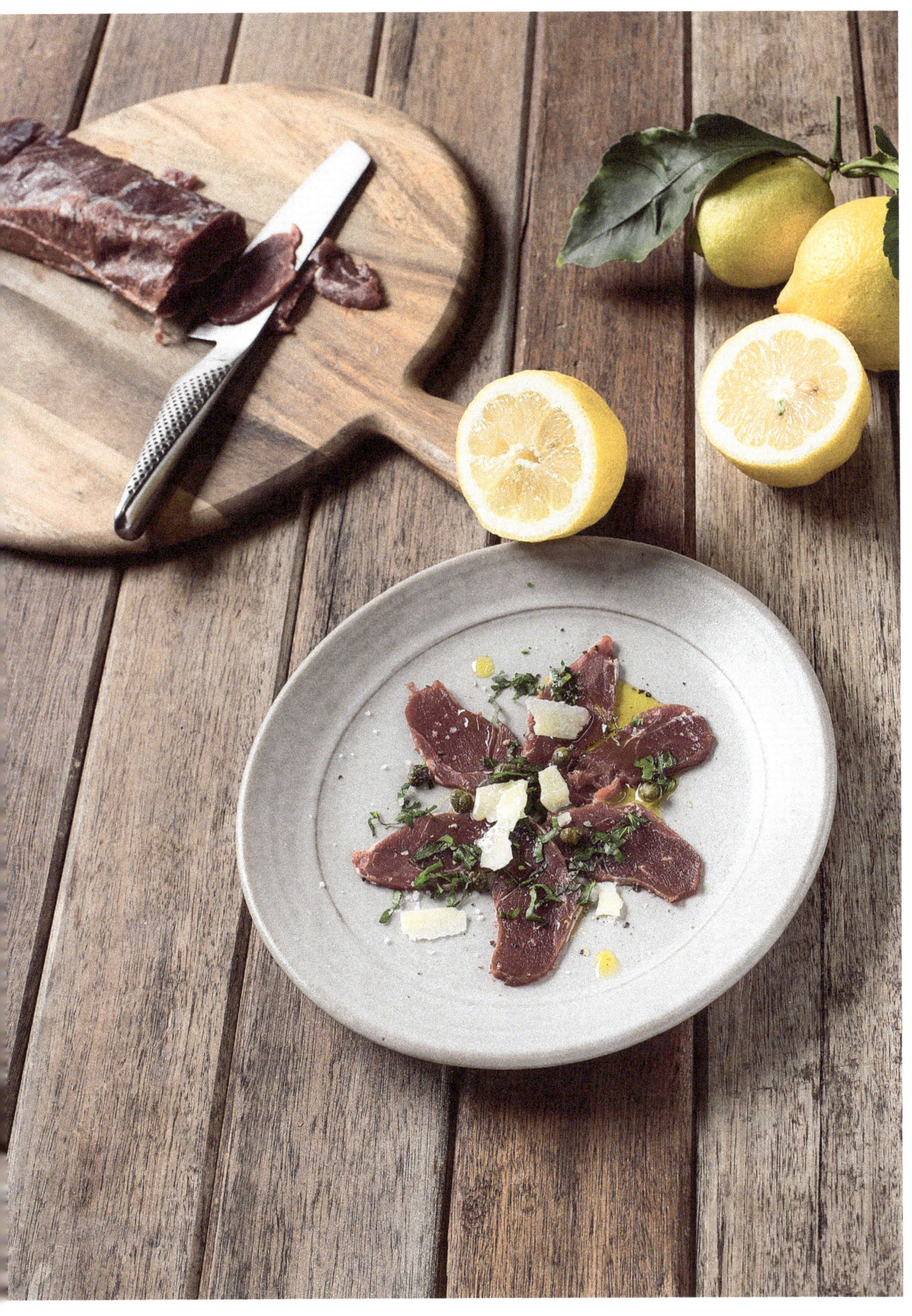

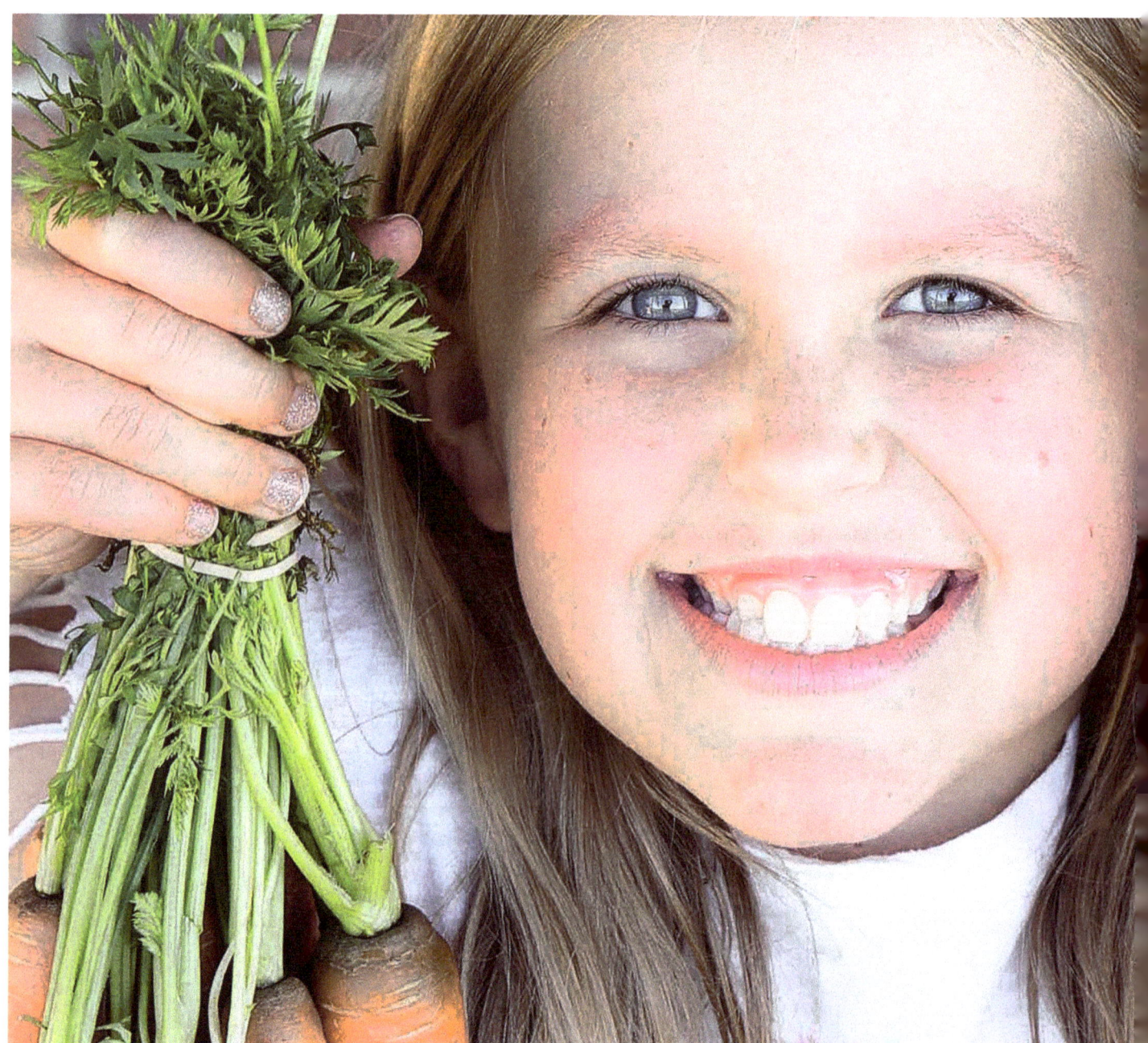

From the Patch

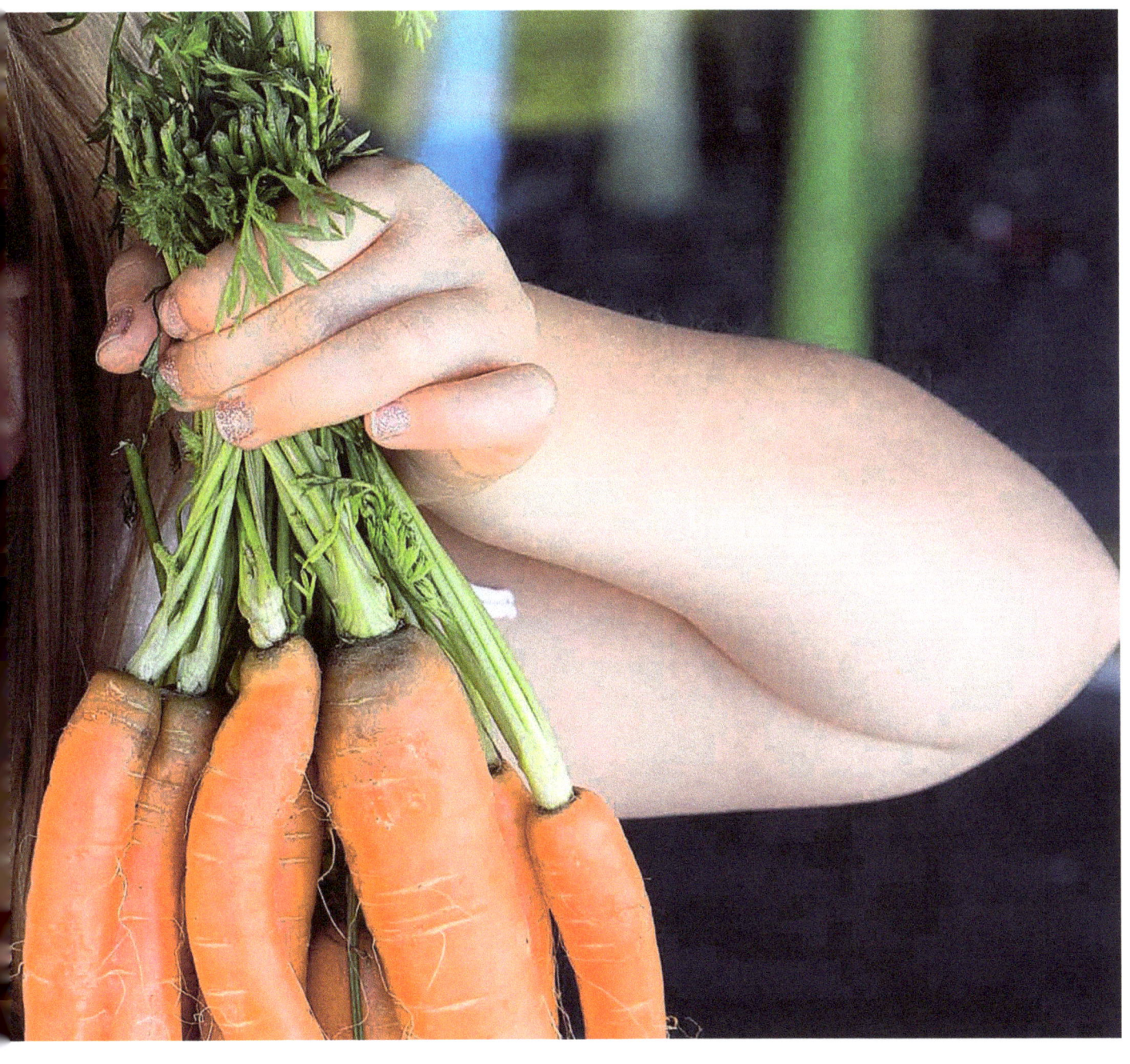

Tomato Sauce

MAKES 8 LITRES

Summer tomatoes in Tasmania taste amazing. Growing a just a few plants is very rewarding - even if they are just in pots on the deck. If you only preserve one thing a year, make it a batch of tomato sauce. This recipe makes 8 litres, so plenty to go around! Halve the quantity if you would like to make less. This sauce is delicious on all savoury foods.

1 kilogram onions

2 bulbs garlic

1 kilogram apples

6 kilograms of tomatoes

1 tablespoon pepper

30 grams salt

½ tablespoon cloves

½ tablespoon mustard powder

1 tablespoon cumin

½ tablespoon chilli

1 cup brown vinegar

1 cup white vinegar

750 grams sugar

Peel and chop the onions and garlic, core and chop the apple and roughly chop the tomatoes. Tip all the ingredients, except for the sugar, into a very large, heavy-based saucepan. Bring to a gentle boil, reduce the heat and simmer for 25 minutes.

Blend well with a stick blender and add the sugar. Simmer for another hour. To test whether the sauce has reached setting point, put a teaspoon on a saucer and put into the fridge for a few minutes – it should have the desired sauce consistency (if not, cook for a few minutes more and then test again).

Pour into hot, sterilized jars, cover and seal.

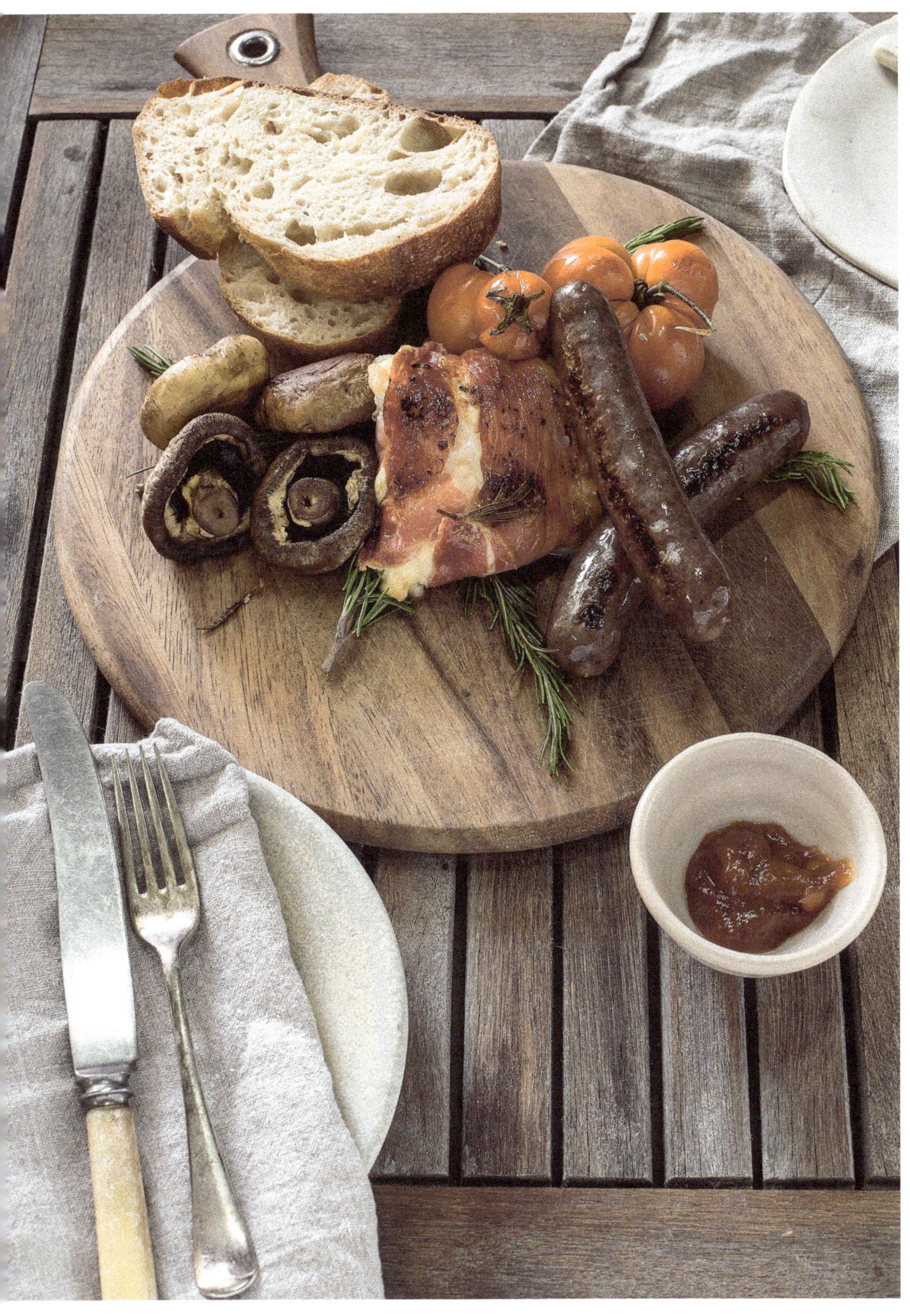

Quinoa, Broccoli and Sundried Tomato Salad

SERVES 4

Quinoa is a grain high in protein and has a lovely, nutty flavour. Most quinoa is imported, however Kindred Organics are a Tasmanian producer - so look out for that brand when you are shopping. This salad is full of flavour and is delicious served with grilled or barbecued meats.

½ cup quinoa

1 head broccoli

1 clove crushed garlic

2 tablespoons extra virgin olive oil

1 tablespoons balsamic vinegar

1 red capsicum

3 tablespoons sundried tomatoes

2 cups spinach leaves

½ bunch basil

Wash the quinoa well by tipping into a large bowl and filling with cold water. Stir a few times and then drain through a sieve. Repeat the process until the water runs clear (some quinoa brands come already washed – just look at the packet to check).

To cook the quinoa, place into a small saucepan with one cup of cold water, bring to the boil, reduce the heat and simmer for approximately 15 minutes or until the grains are tender and water has been absorbed. Fluff with a fork and place in the fridge to cool.

To cook the broccoli, cut small florets of broccoli from the head. Prepare a bowl of iced water. Bring a small saucepan of water to the boil and blanch the florets for 2 minutes, or until just cooked but still bright green and crisp. Plunge into iced water to cool and stop the cooking process, then drain.

To make the salad, crush the garlic and mix with the olive oil and balsamic vinegar in a large bowl. Dice the capsicum, finely chop the sundried tomatoes and spinach and shred the basil. Toss the quinoa, broccoli florets, capsicum, tomatoes, spinach and basil through the dressing and serve.

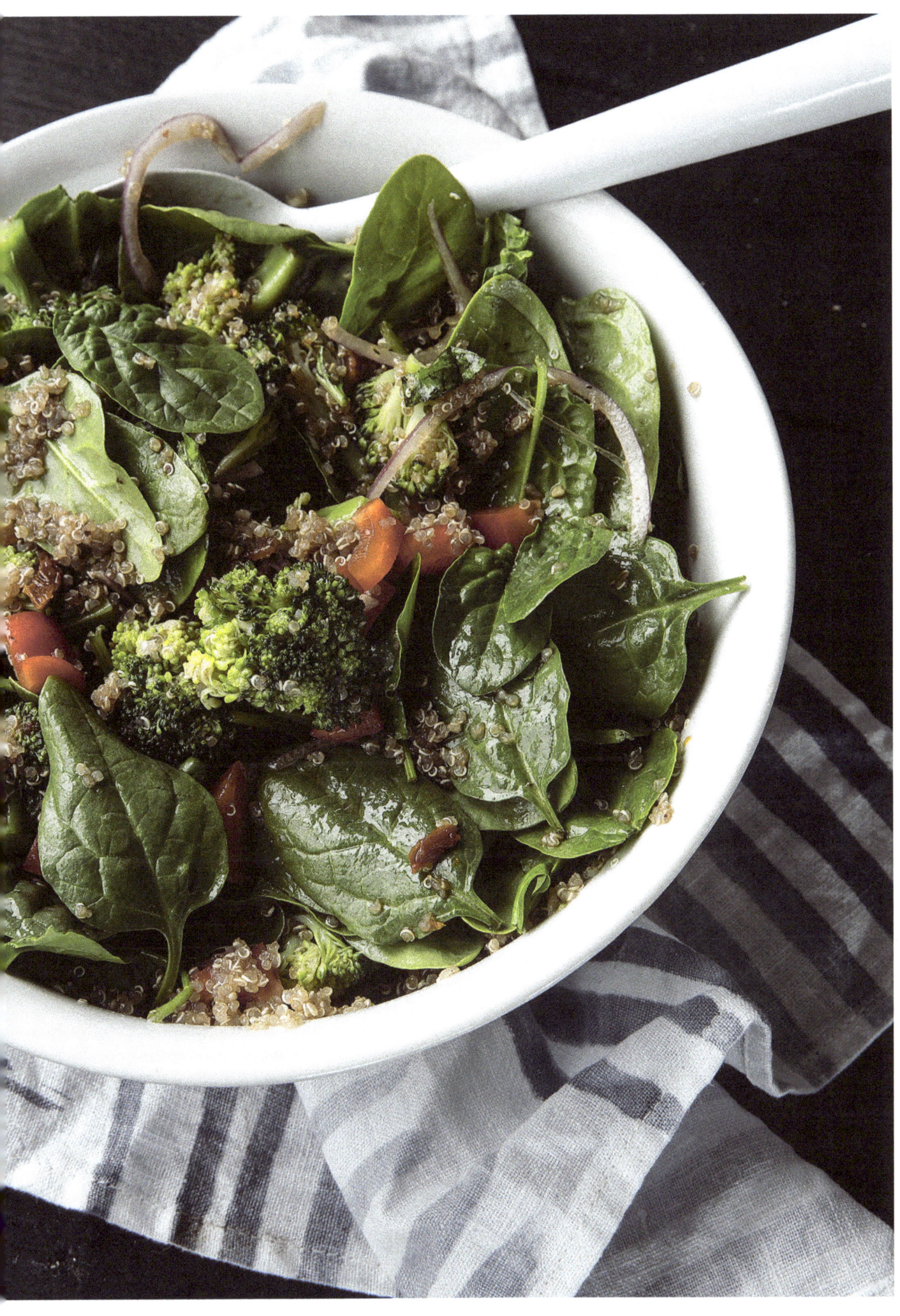

Smoked Salmon and Fennel Salad

SERVES 4

This is a super simple (but very tasty) salad to whip up for a weekday meal or a special occasion.

1 cup peas

1 baby fennel bulb

1 small red onion

½ bunch dill

100 grams feta cheese

3 tablespoons mayonnaise

3 cups spinach leaves

200 grams smoked salmon

To blanch the peas, bring a small saucepan of water to the boil, drop in the peas and cook for one minute. Drain and set aside to cool.

Finely slice the fennel bulb and red onion, and finely chop the dill. Mix together with the peas, crumbled feta, mayonnaise, spinach and fennel. Arrange on a serving platter and top with the smoked salmon.

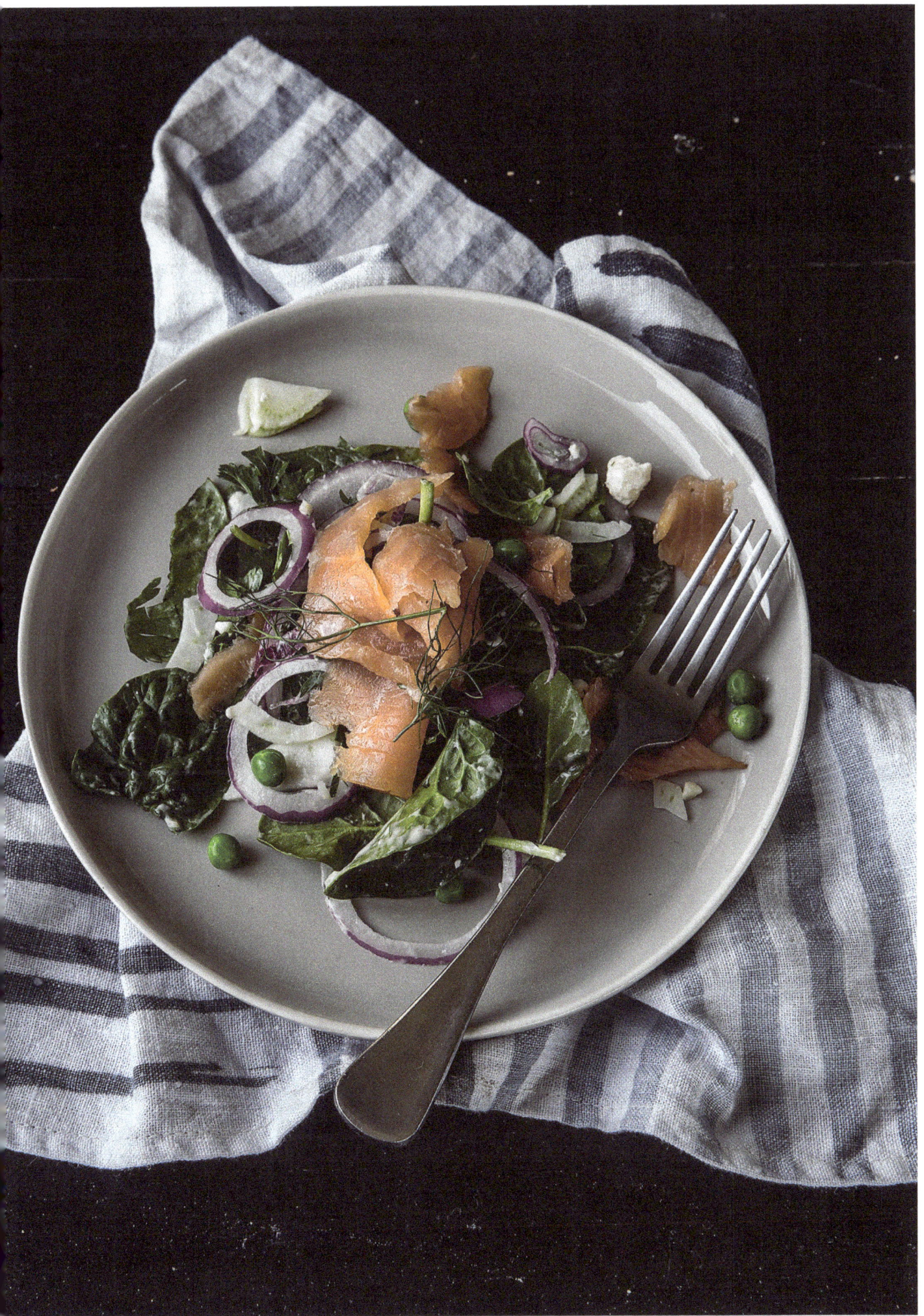

Rhubarb and Custard Tart

SERVES 8

This combination of crisp pastry, creamy custard and tart rhubarb is so delicious. To save time, you could use a food processor to make the base – simply process the cubed butter, flour and sugar, add the egg and enough cold water to bring the dough together. For best results, use a pie tin with a removable base and cover the base with baking paper.

RHUBARB TOPPING

8 stalks rhubarb

1 tablespoon sugar

1-2 teaspoons cold water

CRUST

melted butter and plain flour for preparing the tin

100 grams butter

1 ½ cups plain flour

2 tablespoons sugar

1 egg

PASTRY CREAM FILLING

320ml milk

1 teaspoon vanilla essence

3 egg yolks

2 tablespoons plain flour

2 tablespoons cornflour

2 tablespoons sugar

To stew the rhubarb, cut the stems into 2cm lengths, and place into a heavy-based saucepan with the sugar and water. Bring to a gentle simmer over low heat, cover and continue to simmer for 10 minutes, or until the rhubarb is cooked through but still holds its shape. Remove from the heat and refrigerate until cool. If you prefer, the rhubarb can be cooked for a few minutes more to create a soft puree.

To make the crust, preheat the oven to 180°C. Brush a 20cm pie tin with melted butter and dust with plain flour. Cut the cold butter into small cubes and place in a large bowl with the flour and sugar. Using your fingertips, rub the butter into the flour and sugar until the mixture resembles fine breadcrumbs. Add the egg and one tablespoon of water, and knead to a firm dough. Form the dough into a flat disc, wrap in plastic wrap and refrigerate for one hour. Remove from the fridge, roll out to a thickness of approximately 1/2 cm and line the base and sides of the pie tin with the pastry. Bake for approximately 15 minutes, or until the pastry is golden brown. Remove from the oven and set aside to cool.

To make the pastry cream filling, pour the milk and vanilla essence into a saucepan, place over medium heat and slowly bring to the boil. Once it reaches boiling point, remove from the heat and set aside to cool slightly. Using a large mixing bowl, beat the egg yolks, plain flour, cornflour and sugar together, and then slowly whisk in the hot milk until well combined. Return this mixture to the saucepan, and slowly return to the boil over medium heat, stirring continuously with a wooden spoon. Once the mixture is boiling, continue to stir well for one minute until the pastry cream is thick and smooth. Transfer to a bowl and cover the surface of the pastry cream with plastic wrap (to avoid a skin forming) and transfer to the fridge to cool.

To assemble the tart, remove the pastry cream from the fridge and beat well with a wooden spoon to loosen. Spoon into the cooled tart base and top with the cooled rhubarb. Serve with fresh cream.

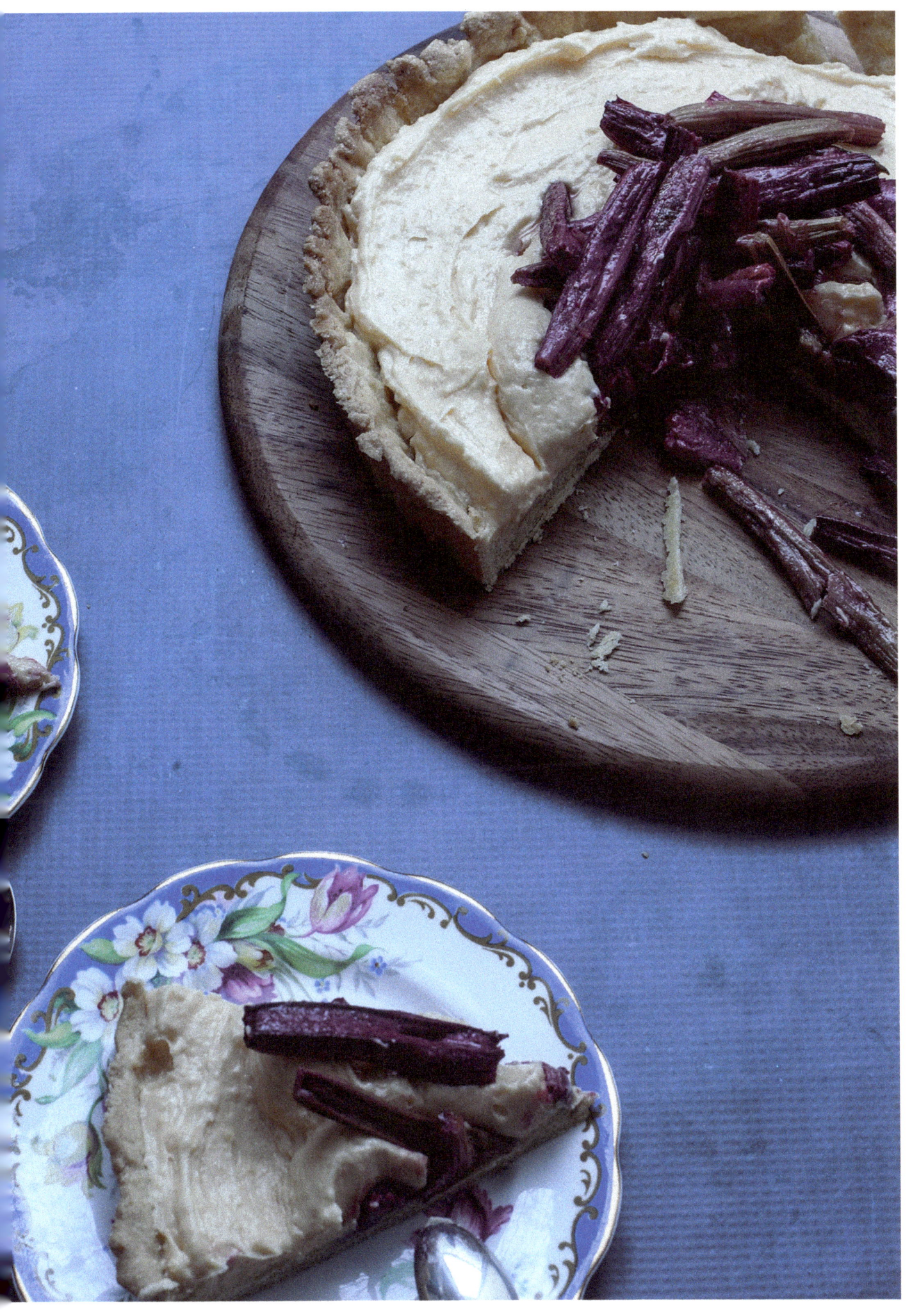

SHAREE MILLS - ENDLESS WAVES HAIRDRESSING

Rustic Country Kitchen Potato Bake

SERVES 6-8

We are so lucky in Tasmania to have access to many different varieties of potatoes – Kennebecs work well in this dish, as do most floury varieties. New season potatoes taste fantastic simply boiled and tossed with butter and fresh herbs, or cooked to use in a summer potato salad. This comforting potato bake is a lovely, warming dish that the whole family will love.

60 grams butter

¼ cup plain flour

⅓ cup milk

2 cups grated tasty cheese

1.2 kilograms Kennebec potatoes

1 cup chicken stock

all purpose seasoning salt

200 grams ham

Preheat the oven to 180°C.

Peel the potatoes and cut into 5mm slices. Slice the ham into thin slices. Melt the butter and whisk it in a bowl with the flour, milk, chicken stock and season with salt and pepper.

Using a ceramic baking dish, lay one third of the potato slices on the bottom of the dish in a thin layer, top with half of the ham and then one third of the cheese.

Add another thin layer of potatoes, remaining ham and another third of the cheese, and finally add the last layer of potatoes. Pour over the milk mixture and sprinkle the last of the cheese on top.

Bake for 30 - 40 minutes or until cooked through and golden.

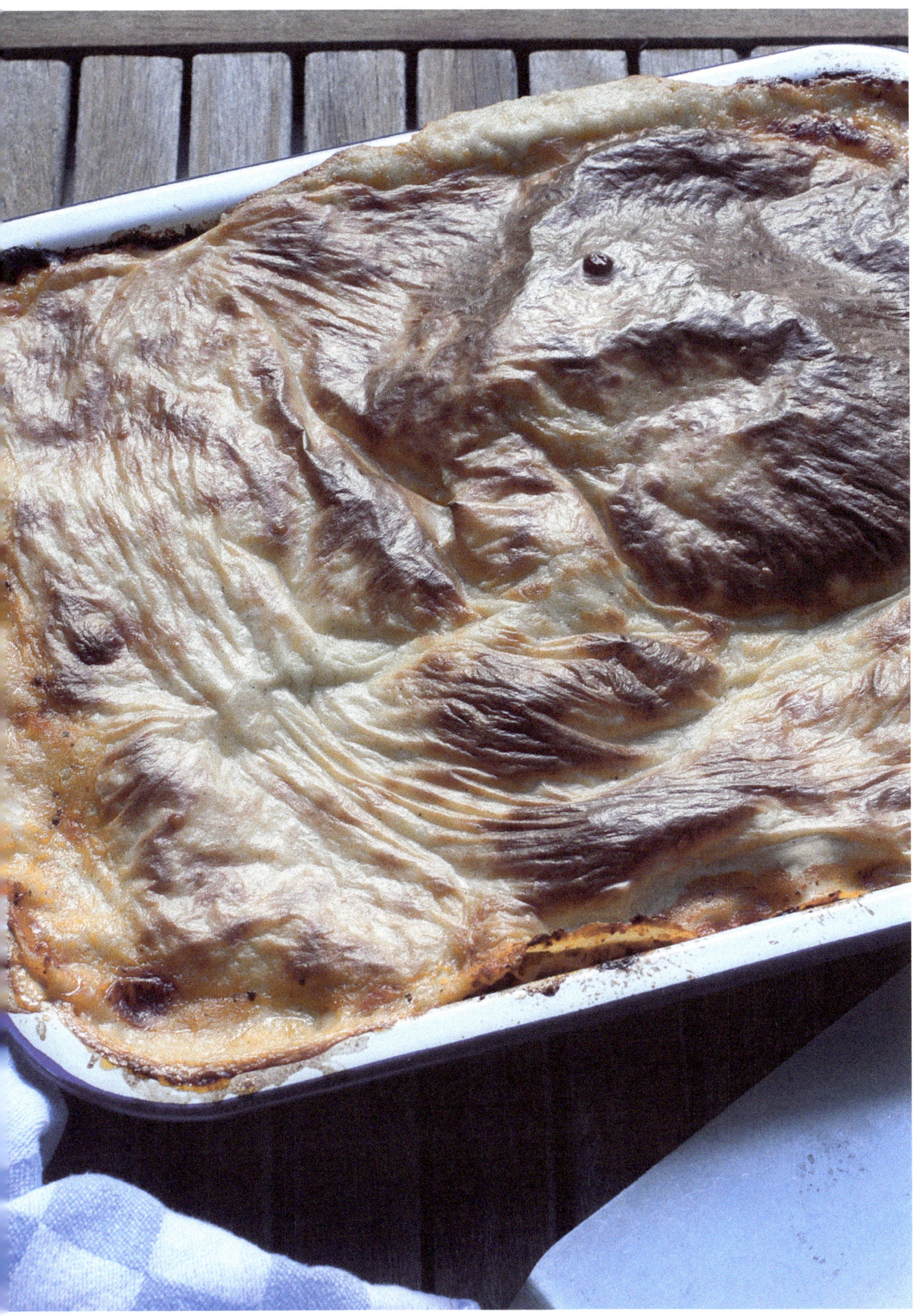

ARWEN GENGE ARWEN'S THERMO PICS

Creamy Potato Salad

SERVES 8-10 AS A SIDE DISH

This potato salad has a lovely creamy dressing, but would be delicious topped with any dressing you choose – try aioli, béarnaise sauce, toum (a Lebanese garlic sauce), French dressing or even simple natural yoghurt or mayonnaise. Pink eye potatoes are seasonally available in Tasmania – substitute any waxy potato.

800 grams pink eye potatoes

6 eggs

6 spring onions and/or chives

½ cup fresh Italian parsley

1 clove garlic

1 teaspoon Dijon or seeded mustard

1 cup sour cream

salt and cracked black pepper

OPTIONAL

3 tablespoons fresh dill

smoked salmon and capers or crispy bacon

To cook the potatoes and eggs, place the potatoes into a saucepan, cover with cold water and bring to the boil. When the water is boiling, add the eggs and cook for 7 minutes, and then remove from the water with a slotted spoon (this will result in eggs with a slightly runny yolk – continue cooking for a further 3 minutes if you prefer a hard boiled egg).

Continue to cook the potatoes for another 10 minutes, or until cooked to your liking. Drain the potatoes and peel the eggs. Set aside to cool. Cut the eggs into quarters and arrange on a serving platter with the potatoes.

To make the dressing, finely chop the spring onions and/or chives, parsley, dill and garlic and set aside. Stir together the mustard and sour cream, mix in the salt and pepper and most of the spring onions and herbs – reserving some to sprinkle on top.

Pour the dressing over the potatoes and eggs and stir gently to combine. Sprinkle with the reserved spring onions and herbs. This potato salad is best served warm but is also delicious cold.

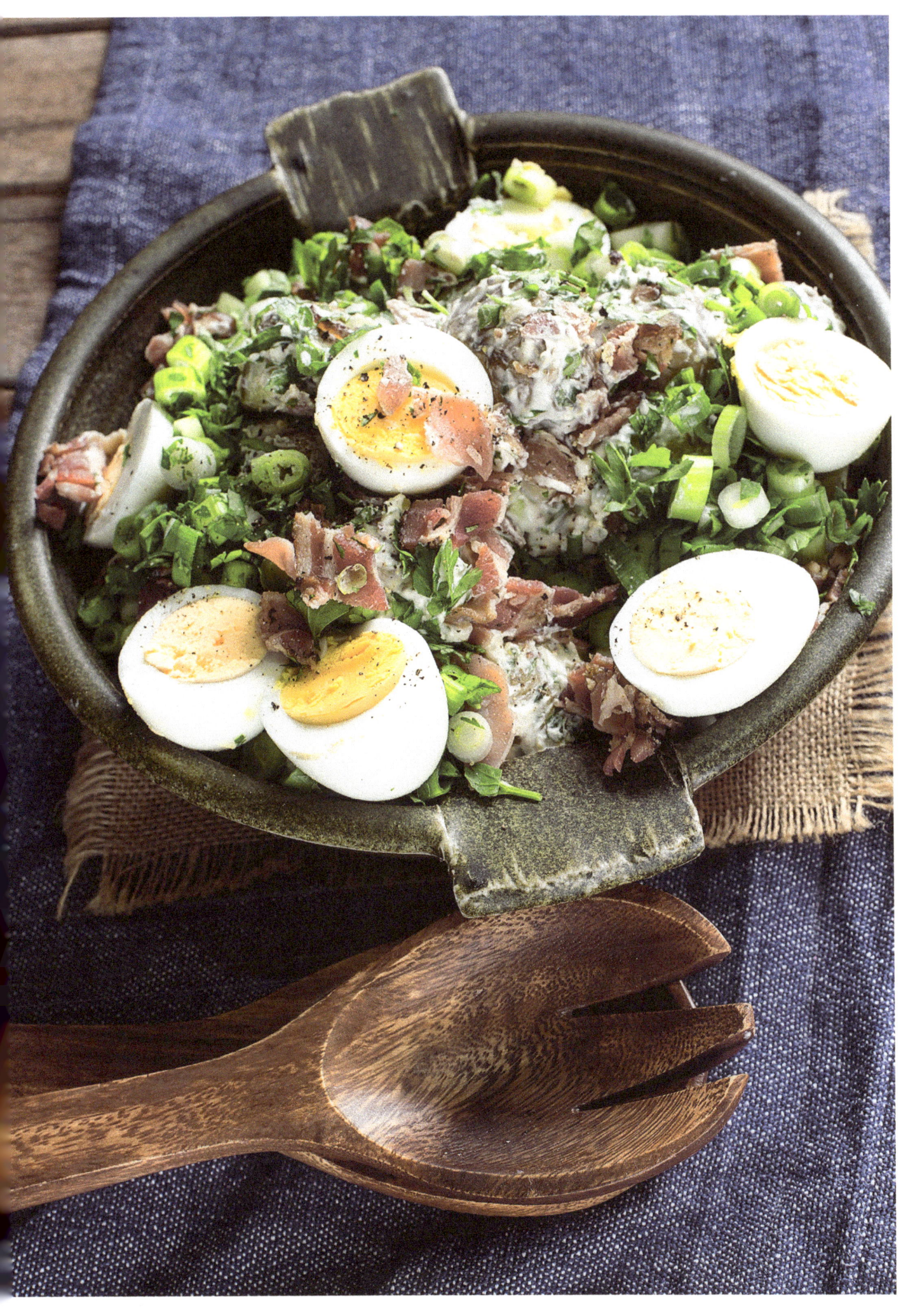

Breakfast Bagel with Ricotta and Balsamic Tomatoes

SERVES 4

This is a lovely option if you are looking for a special occasion breakfast that is a little bit lightern – but it's so quick and easy that it's perfect for any day, really!

200 grams cherry tomatoes

2 tablespoons parsley

2 tablespoons balsamic vinegar

1 tablespoon extra virgin olive oil

50 grams baby spinach or rocket leaves

4 bagels

100 grams light ricotta cheese

sea salt and cracked pepper

Make the tomato mix by halving the tomatoes, and roughly chopping the parsley. Combine the tomatoes and parsley in a bowl with balsamic vinegar, extra virgin olive oil, spinach or rocket and toss well to combine.

Cut the bagels in half, lightly toast and spread with the ricotta cheese. Top with the tomato mix, season with salt and pepper and serve.

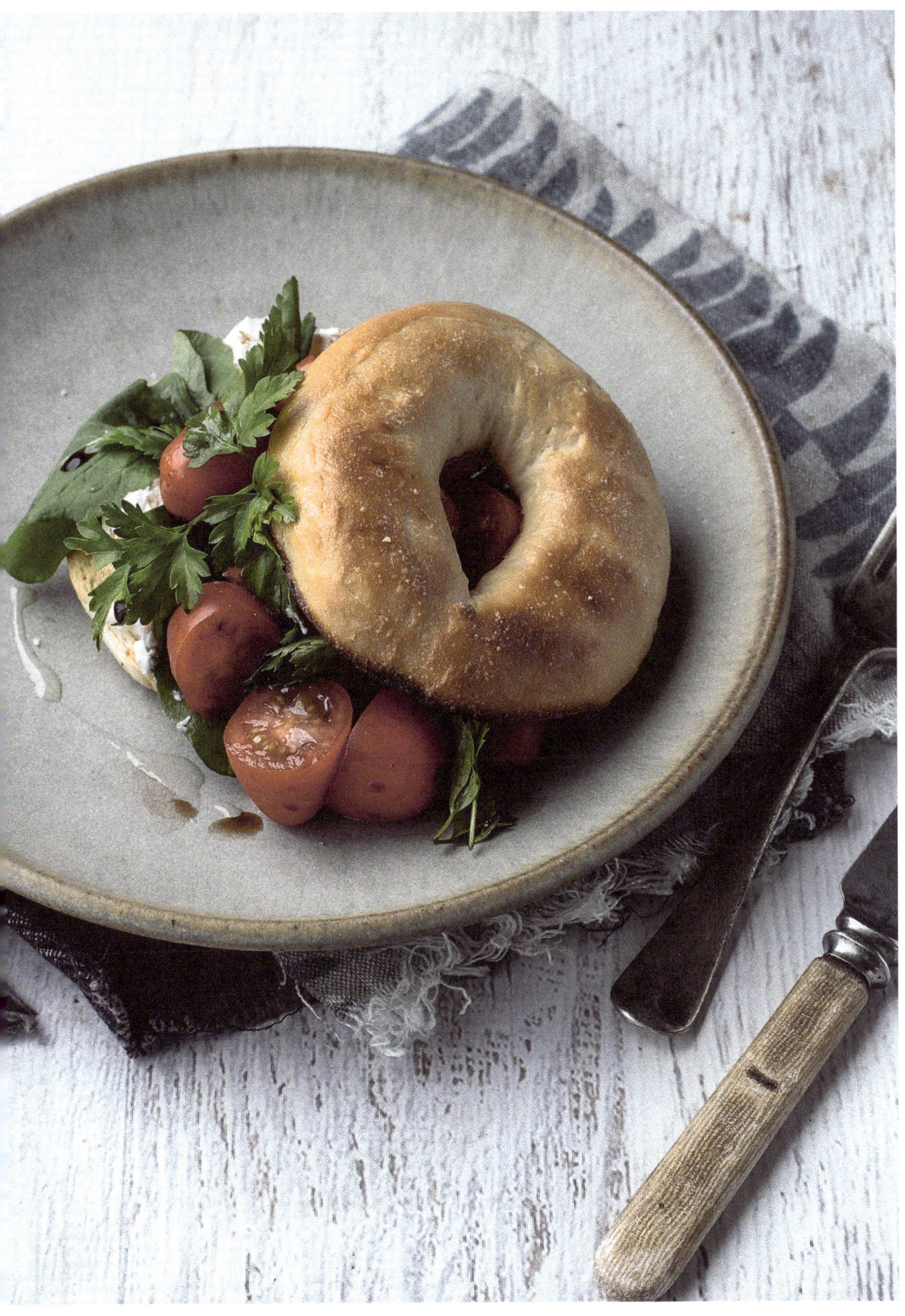

Fermented Honey Garlic

MAKES ONE JAR

Fermented honey garlic is a wonderful natural remedy for colds and flu and is also delicious used in marinades, as a glaze for meat or in any savoury recipe calling for honey. This is a very simple method and can be easily scaled up if necessary, if you would like to make a larger quantity.

3 bulbs of garlic

raw honey

Separate the garlic into individual cloves and peel each clove. Tip garlic cloves into a glass jar and pour over honey until all cloves are well covered. Loosely cover the jar with a lid to allow the gasses to escape.

Place the jar on a saucer and store in a cool, dark place and allow to ferment for two weeks, turning the jar over every few days to ensure the garlic and honey are well mixed. The garlic will darken and honey will become runnier over time, with the garlic becoming milder in flavour as it develops.

Store in a cool, dark place.

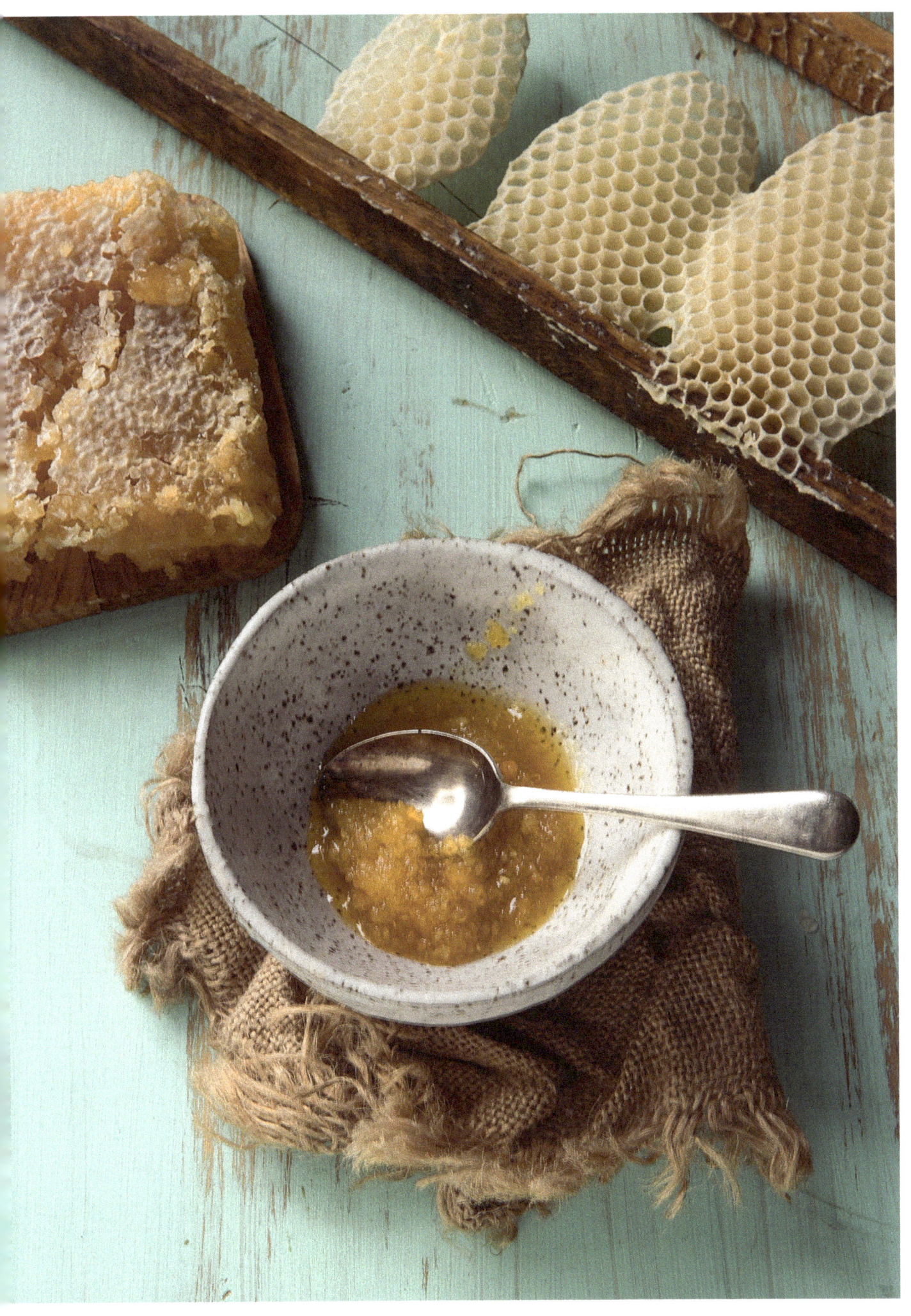

PENNI LAMPREY - BEE PATIENT HONEY

Fermented Seeded Mustard

MAKES 400G

This delicious mustard goes with everything – chunks of ham, grilled pork loins, creamy sauces, in salad dressings and lots more. Using whey helps to kick start the fermentation process, and fermenting the mustard both preserves it and makes more nutrients available. If you like to make your own cheese you can use they whey from this process, or simply strain some good quality natural yoghurt through cheesecloth to collect the whey. This recipe can be easily doubled and combined in a food processor to create a smooth paste if you prefer.

70 grams yellow mustard seeds

70 grams brown mustard seeds

2 teaspoons dry mustard powder

50ml whey (optional)

2 teaspoons of sea salt

85 grams raw honey

120ml water

Combine all the ingredients together in a bowl, and mix very well to ensure the ingredients are very well incorporated. Transfer to a glass jar and secure with a tight fitting lid. Store in a cool, dark place at room temperature for 3-5 days, tasting each day.

Once the taste is to your liking, store the jar in the fridge and use as required.

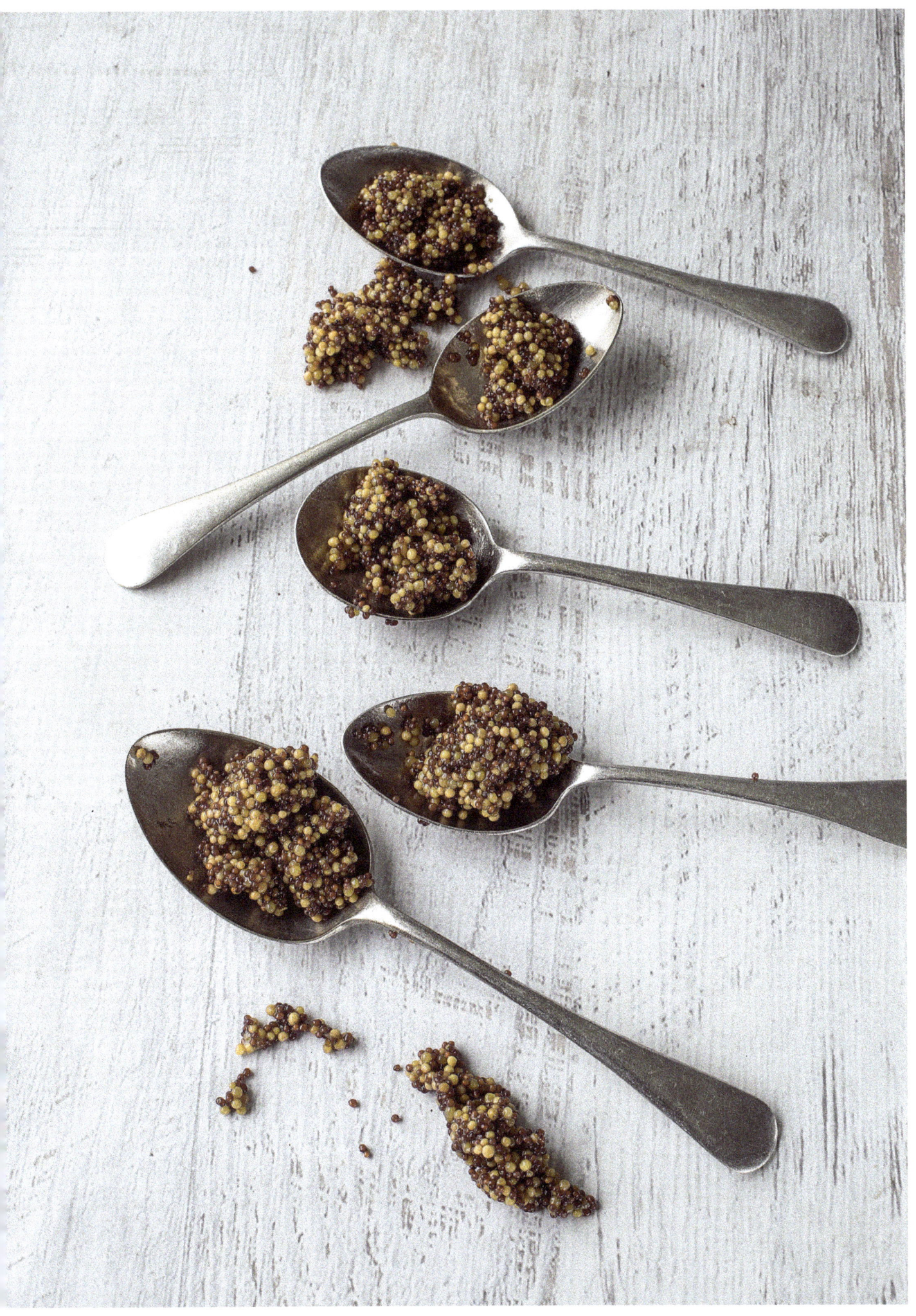

Summer Berry Pudding

SERVES 6

Any combination of summer berries can be used in this glorious dessert, and it really looks its best when layered in a straight sided glass dish – although you can also make individual servings in smaller glasses or ramekins. Omit the Cointreau for an alcohol free dessert.

125 grams caster sugar

2 tablespoons of lemon juice

100ml water

90ml Cointreau

3 punnets berries

250 grams cream cheese

150ml cream

2 tablespoons icing sugar

1 teaspoon vanilla essence

1 teaspoon vanilla essence

200 grams sponge fingers

Make a syrup by heating the sugar, lemon juice and water in a saucepan over medium heat, bring to the boil, reduce heat and simmer until the sugar has dissolved, then add the Cointreau. Set aside to cool slightly and then add the berries to the warm syrup.

Using a food processor, blend the softened cream cheese, cream, icing sugar and vanilla until smooth.

Cover the bottom of a large, glass bowl with sponge finger biscuits, top with a generous layer of the cream mixture and spoon over some of the berry syrup. Continue layering in this manner.

Refrigerate for a few hours or overnight before serving.

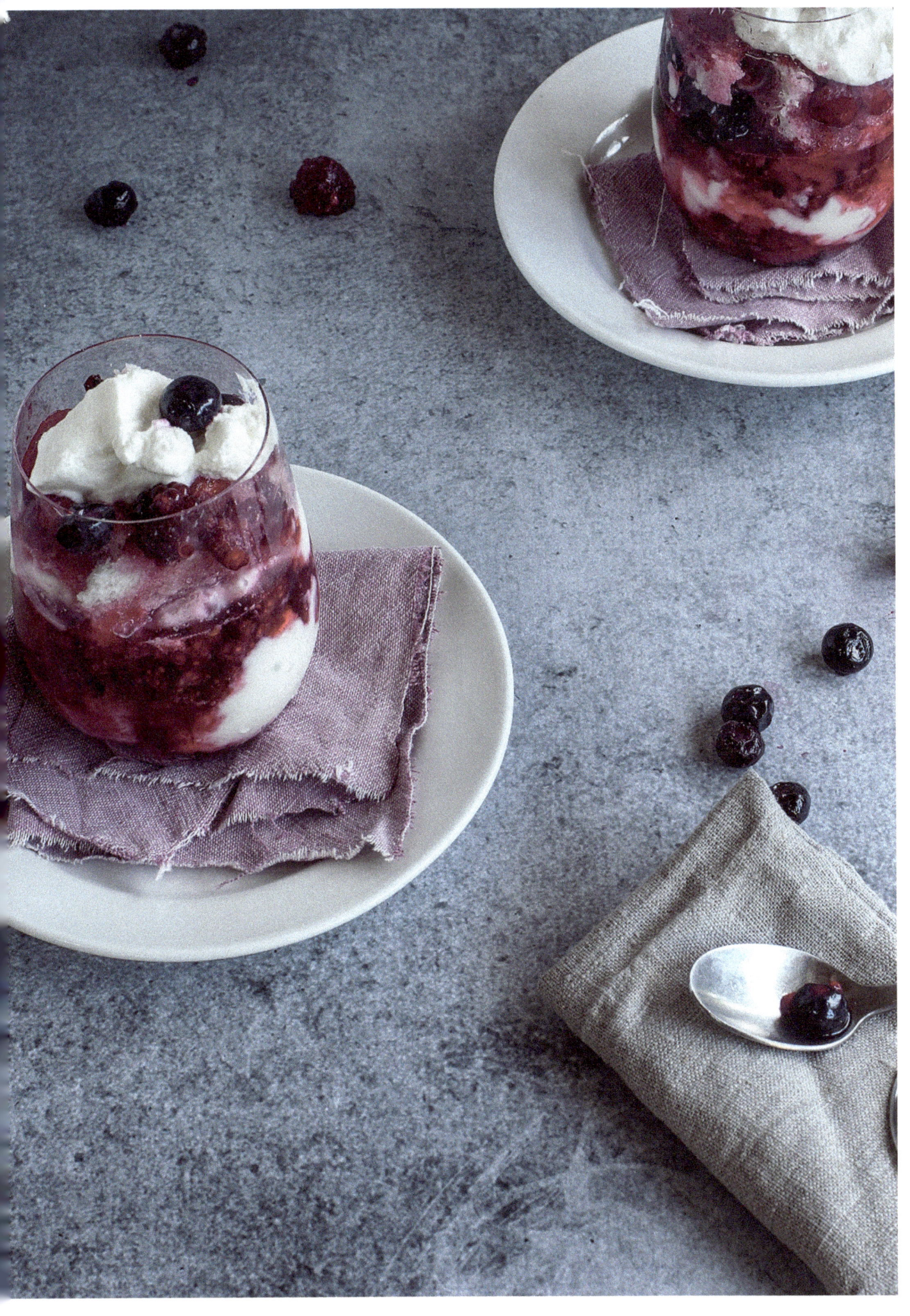

Roast Tomato and Roast Garlic Soup

SERVES 4

Roasting the vegetables for this soup brings out their sweet flavours - add the cream to create a lovely rich soup, or leave it out for something a little bit lighter. Serve with crusty bread and butter.

1 bulb garlic

1 onion

1 kilogram tomatoes

1 tablespoon fresh basil

1 tablespoon fresh oregano

2 tablespoons extra virgin olive oil

1 litre chicken stock

salt and pepper

100ml cream (optional)

Preheat the oven to 180°C.

Separate the garlic into cloves and peel the skin off each one, then roughly chop the onion, and halve the tomatoes. Place the garlic, onion, basil and oregano into a baking tray, drizzle with the extra virgin olive oil and season well with salt and pepper. Put into the oven and cook for 20 minutes or until the vegetables are tender and golden.

Transfer the contents of the baking tray to a heavy-based saucepan and add the stock. Bring to the boil over medium heat, simmer for 10 minutes, remove from the heat and puree using a stick mixer.

Season with salt and pepper and add cream if you wish.

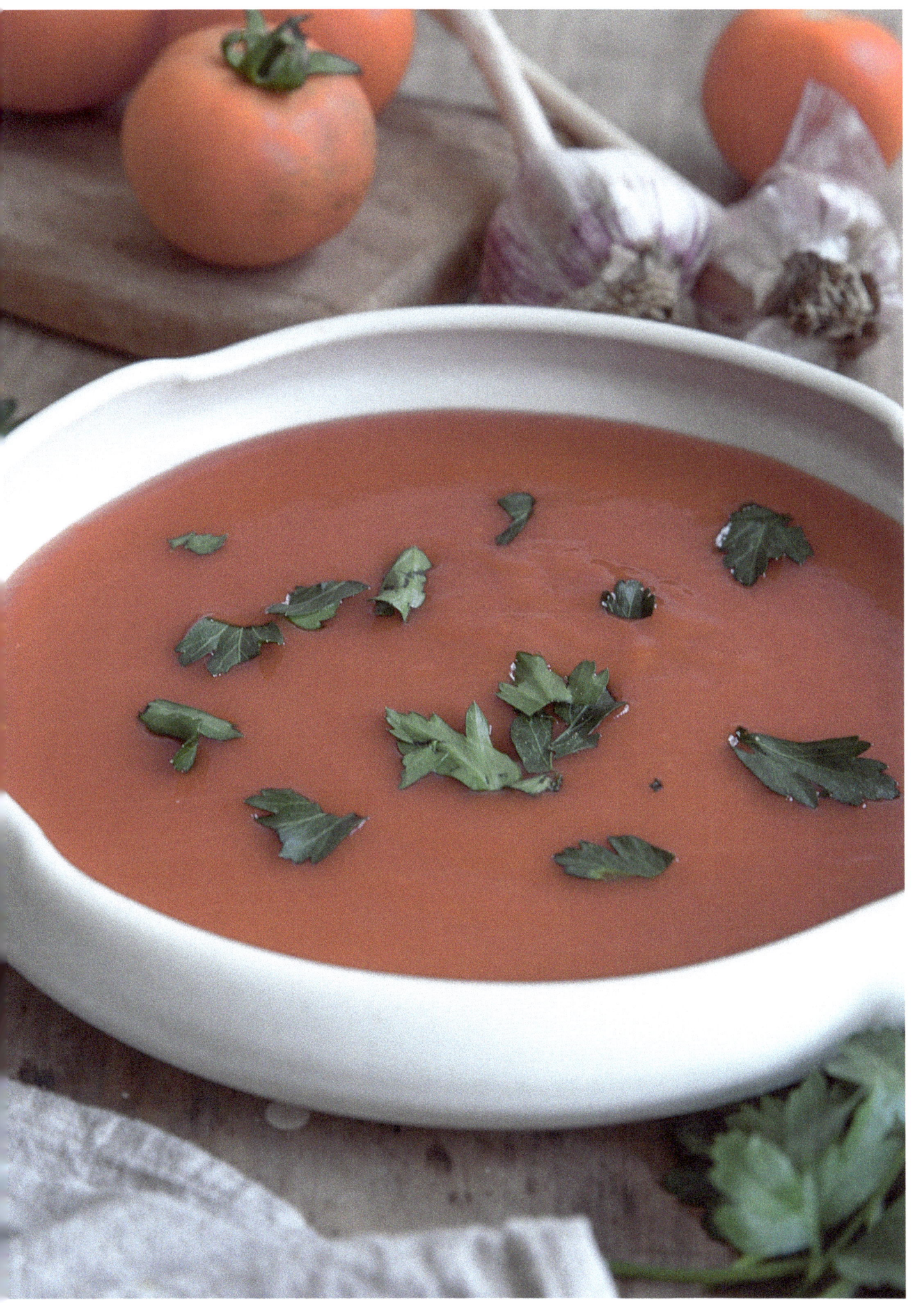

Easy Strawberry Jam

MAKES 6 X 300ML JARS

There are a number of berry farms in Tasmania, and picking your own strawberries is a lovely activity to do with children. This strawberry jam is fabulous with scones, jam and cream, as a filling for a sponge cake – or simply on hot buttered toast. The apple and lemons contain pectin which will help the jam to set – you can grate them using the large holes on a box grater or quickly blitz in the food processor. This simple jam is suitable for stone fruit as well as other berries.

Visit my website eloiseemmett.com to find the recipe to make Monte Carlos, and making these biscuits is such a fun activity to entertain the kids.

1 kilogram strawberries

1 lemon

2 apples

1 kilogram sugar

Remove the stems from the strawberries, grate the whole lemon and apples (including the skin and the pips) and tip all of the fruit into in a large heavy-based saucepan. Pour in 2 cups of cold water and bring this mixture to the boil over medium heat.

Reduce to a simmer and cook for approximately 25 minutes, until the fruit is soft. Remove from the heat and puree with a stick mixer. Add the sugar to the saucepan, return to the boil and simmer until the jam reaches setting point – this will take approximately 30 minutes to one hour.

To check the setting point, dollop some jam onto a cold saucer and put into the fridge for a minute or two, take it out and check if it is set. If so, remove the jam from the heat. If not, continue to simmer for a few more minutes before testing again.

Pour into clean, sterilised jars and store in a cool, dark place.

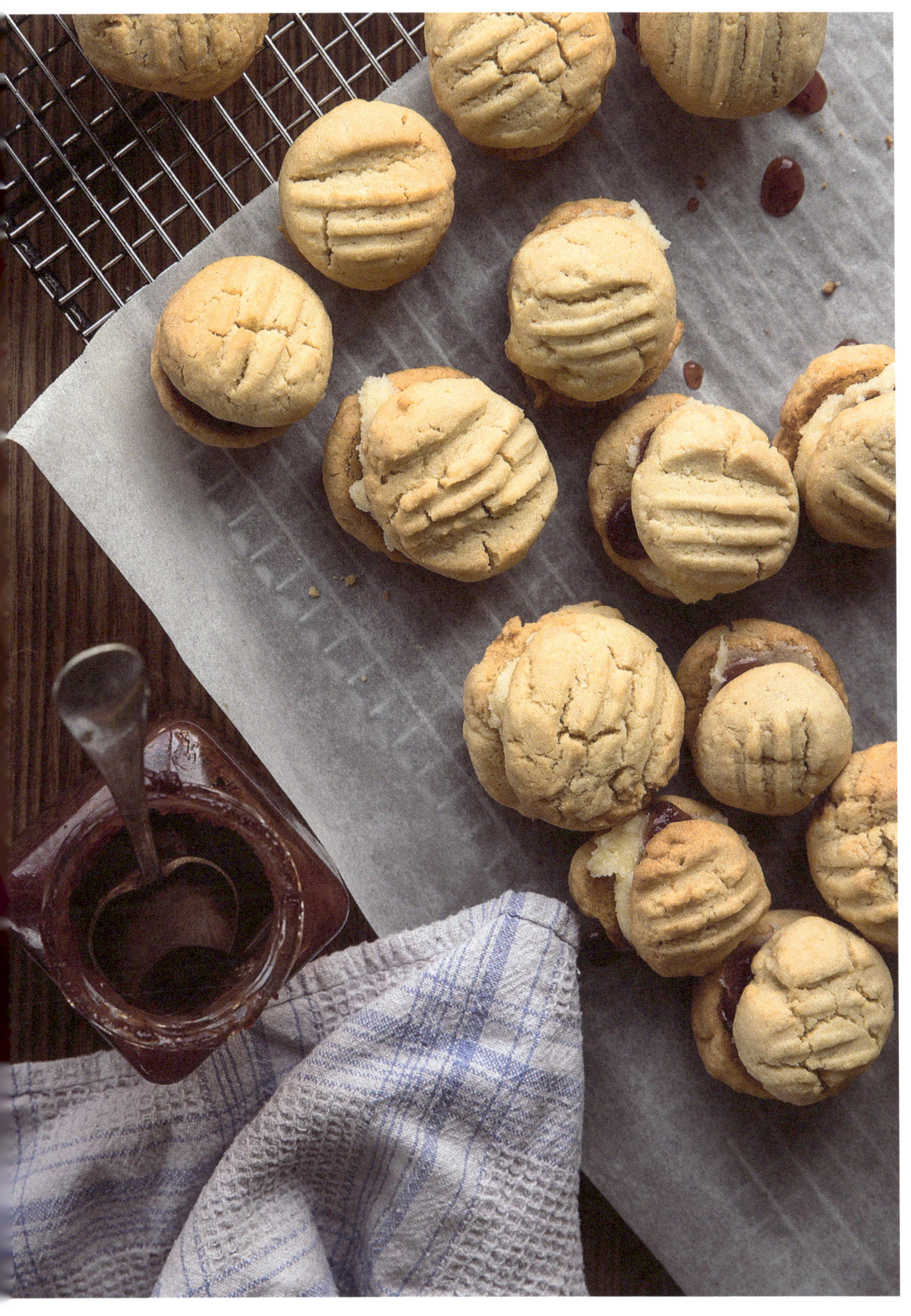

Pumpkin, Cauliflower and Red Lentil Dahl

SERVES 4

This is a very quick and nutritious dinner, and my kids love it! I leave the chilli out when making it for them, but you can add some finely chopped chilli to your own dish if you like a bit of extra heat. This freezes well so I always have a container or two ready for a quick and healthy meal on a busy night.

2cm piece ginger

2 cloves garlic

1 onion

1 red capsicum

1 large carrot

1 teaspoon extra virgin olive oil

200 grams pumpkin

1 ½ cups cauliflower florets

1 cup red lentils

1 cup water

20 grams palm sugar

1 teaspoon garam masala

½ teaspoon mustard seeds

1 teaspoon ground coriander

½ a red chilli

200ml coconut milk

400 grams crushed tomatoes

juice of ½ lemon

salt and pepper

Crush garlic and ginger, and finely dice the onion, capsicum and carrot. Heat a large, heavy-based saucepan over medium heat, add the oil and sauté the garlic, ginger, onion, capsicum and carrot for 5 minutes or until the vegetables have softened.

Chop the pumpkin and cauliflower into 1cm dice and add to the saucepan, along with all of the remaining ingredients and season with salt and pepper. Bring to the boil, reduce the heat and simmer for approximately 20 minutes, or until the vegetables are cooked.

After this time, the pumpkin and cauliflower will be soft and well cooked – if you prefer them with a little more texture, add the pumpkin after 10 minutes of cooking time, and the cauliflower after 15 minutes.

Serve the Dahl with naan bread or some wraps for dipping, and natural yogurt on the side.

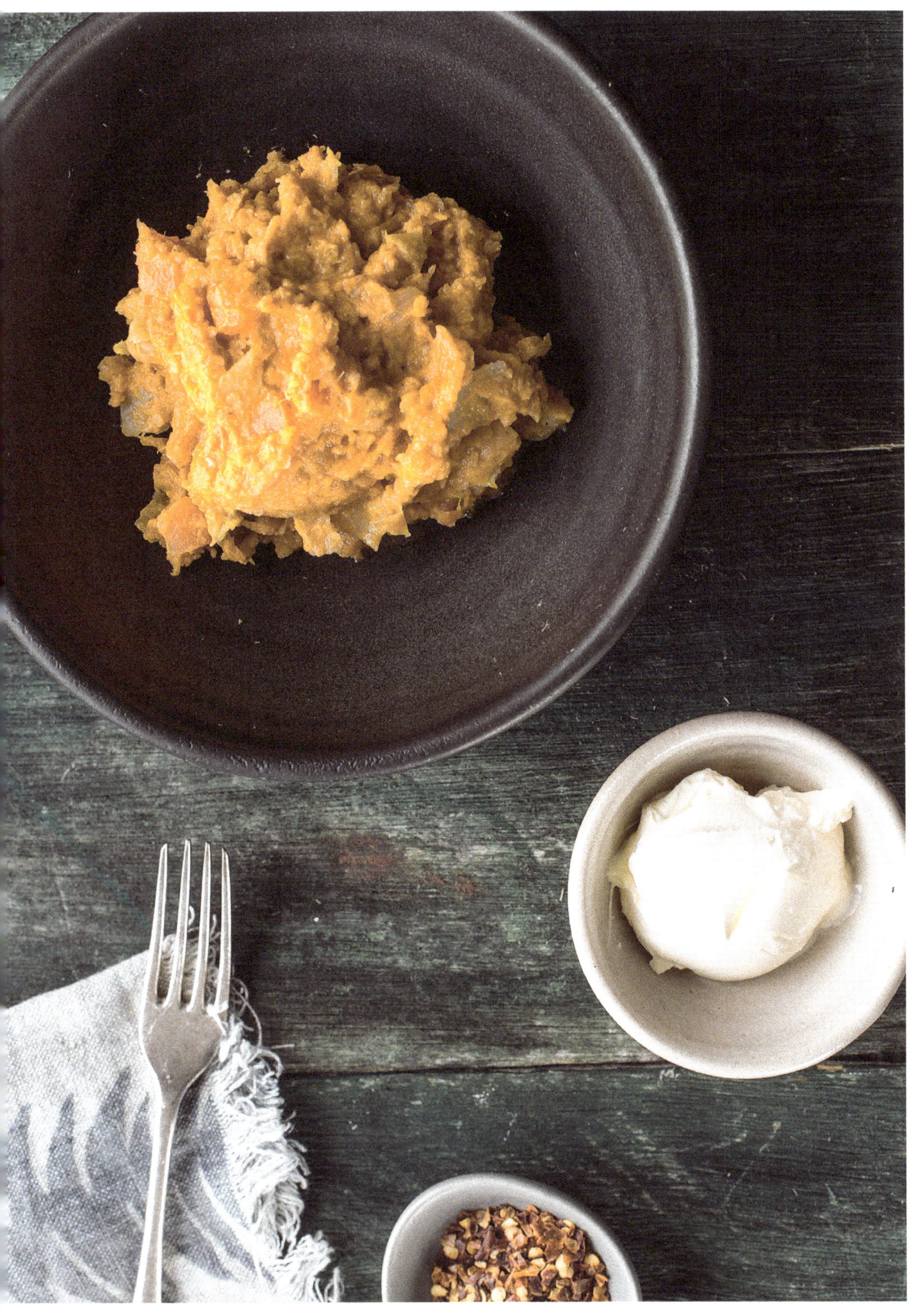

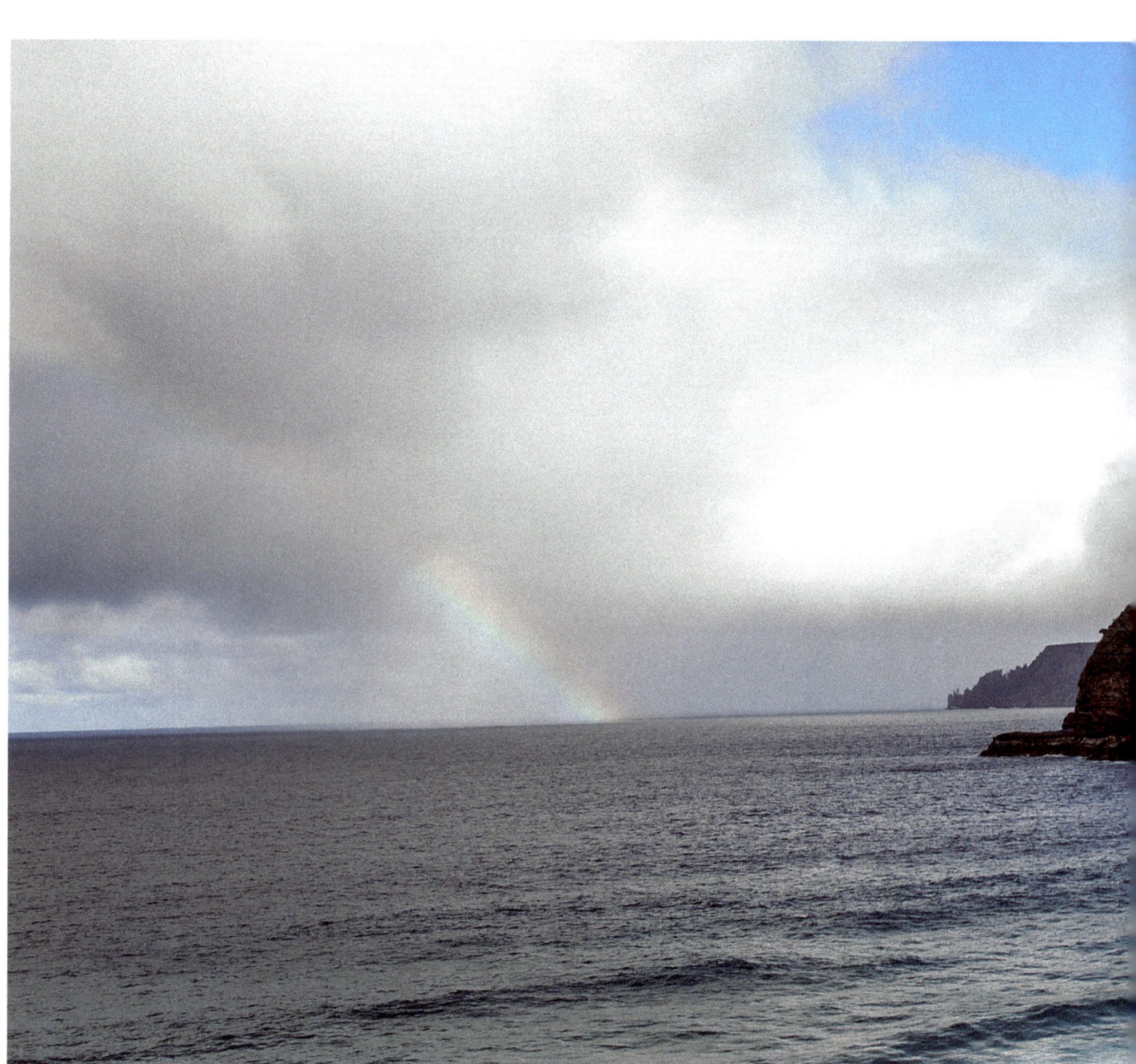

Wild Caught from the Ocean

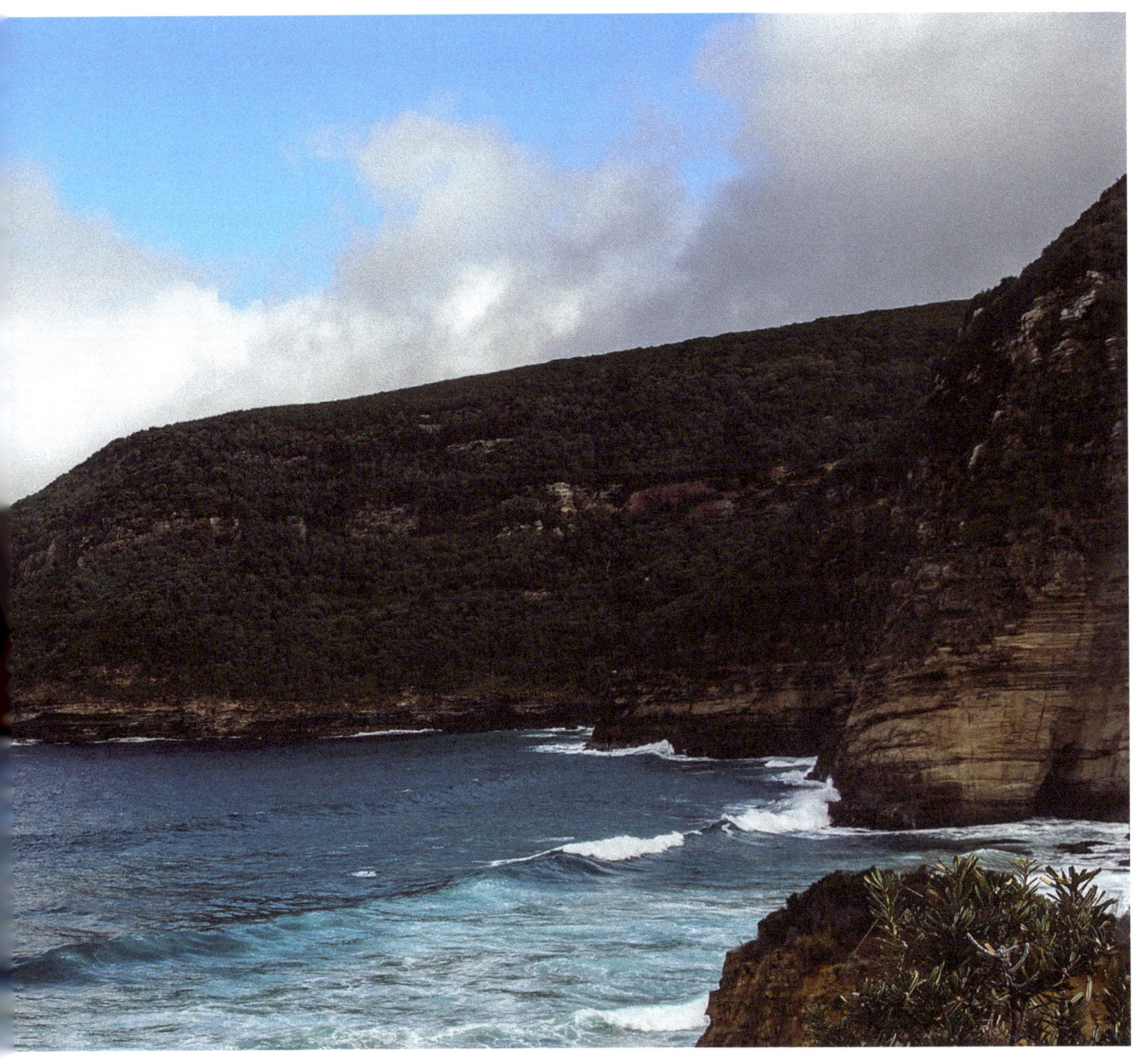

King Island Baked Octopus

SERVES 8

This is a traditional Portuguese recipe, known as Polvo a Lagareiro. It is a good idea to freeze your octopus – this helps with the tenderisation process, simply defrost before cooking. The octopus is delicious served with Portuguese 'punched' potatoes – roast small potatoes with their skins on and once cooked through and soft, wrap your hand in a tea towel and use your fist to 'punch' or crush the potatoes to make them pop open. Drizzle the potatoes with garlic oil to serve.

1 or 2 small octopus (2 kilograms each)
3 onions
5 cloves garlic
2 bay leaves
extra virgin olive oil (enough to cover octopus)
salt and pepper

Bring a large saucepan of water to a simmer and cook the octopus in the water for 15 minutes. Remove from heat and plunge the octopus into iced water to stop the cooking process, then drain well.

Preheat the oven to 220°C. Slice the onions, finely chop the garlic and tip into a baking dish along with the bay leaves. Place the octopus on top of the onions and pour over enough extra virgin olive oil to almost completely immerse the octopus. Season with salt and pepper and cook in the oven for 30-45 minutes, or until tender and lightly browned on the top.

Serve the octopus with punched potatoes and onions from the baking pan, all drizzled generously with extra virgin olive oil from the pan.

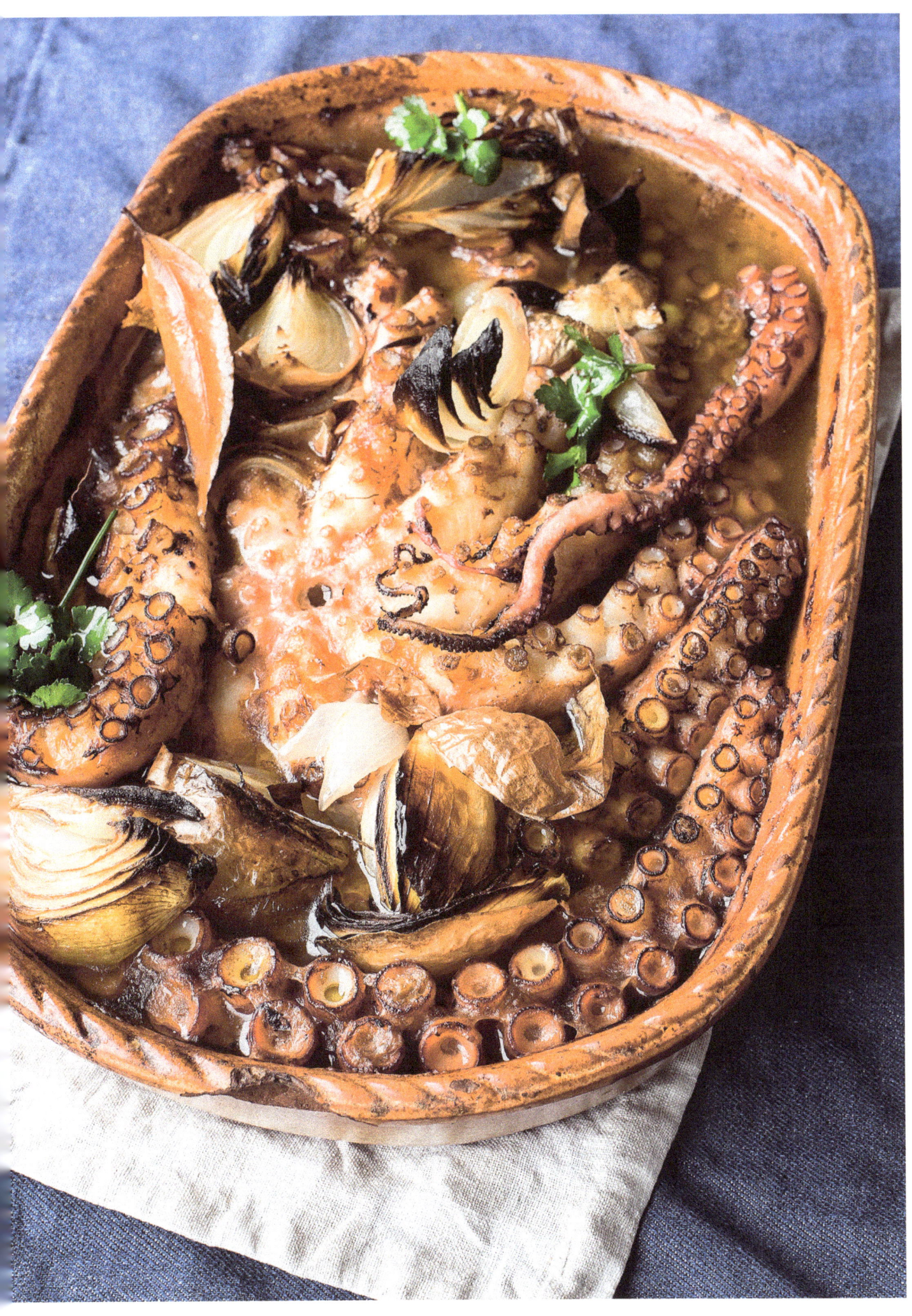

Chili, Lemon and Garlic Squid Fettuccini

SERVES 4

Either squid or calamari can be used for this recipe. If you have caught your own, don't throw the legs away – they are a little bit chewier, but absolutely delicious!

2 onions

4 cloves garlic

2 long red chillies

2 lemons

2 squid-tubes and legs

1 tablespoon extra virgin olive oil

2 tablespoons tarragon

30 grams butter

80 grams Parmesan cheese

1 quantity fresh pasta – see page 158 for the recipe

To make the pasta sauce, peel and slice the onion, and peel and crush the garlic. Cut the chillies in half lengthways, remove the seeds and finely slice. Zest and juice the lemons. Slice the squid into 5mm wide strips. Heat the extra virgin olive oil in a heavy-based frying pan over medium and sauté the garlic and onion for 3 minutes or until softened. Add the squid, chilli, tarragon and butter and and continue to sauté for 5 minutes, or until the squid is just cooked through but not chewy. Cook the pasta, and toss it through the sauce. Serve immediately topped with shaved Parmesan cheese.

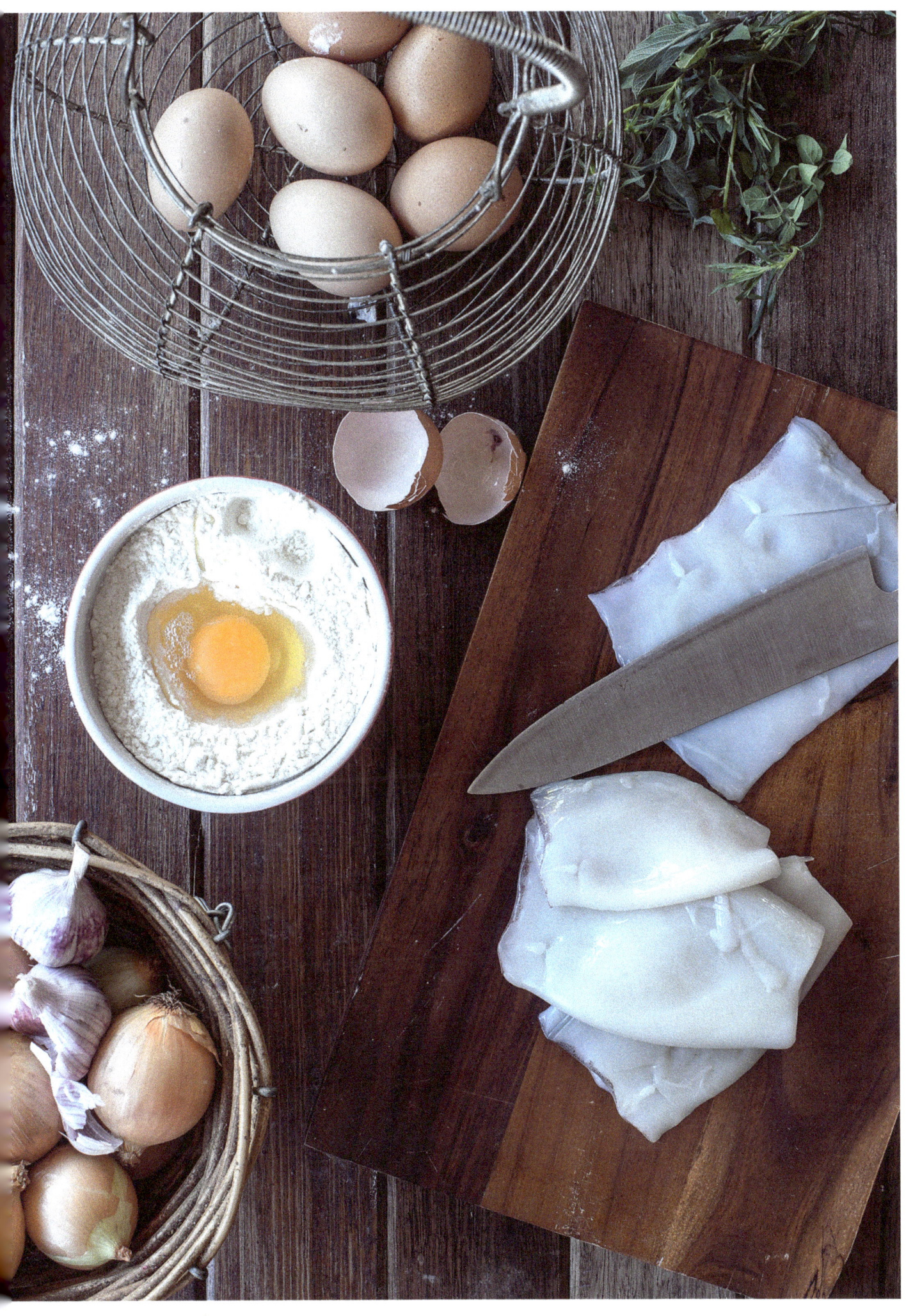

Creamy Crayfish Beef and Reef

SERVES 2

Beef and reef is an absolute classic and so delicious when it's made well! The essential ingredients are a good quality grilling steak (such as eye fillet, scotch fillet or porterhouse), real cream (not a white sauce) and fresh garlic (not out of a jar). Prawns or scallops can be used instead of crayfish. Follow this recipe and you can't go wrong!

1 whole crayfish

1 tablespoon extra virgin olive oil

½ small onion

2 cloves garlic

30ml white wine

200ml cream

1 tablespoon fresh tarragon

sea salt and cracked pepper

2 porterhouse steaks

To cook the crayfish, bring a large pot of salted water to the boil and add the crayfish. When the water returns to the boil, cook for 8 minutes. Drain the crayfish by hanging it over the side of the pot. Cut in half and remove the meat from the tail, body and legs, but leave a few legs to garnish, if you like.

To make the sauce, finely dice the onion and crush the garlic. Heat the oil in a heavy-based pan over low heat, and sauté the garlic and onion for three minutes, or until translucent. Deglaze the pan by pouring in the wine, then add the cream and simmer gently until the sauce thickens. Finely chop the tarragon, add to the sauce and season well with salt and pepper, then toss through the crayfish meat.

To cook your steak, preheat a grill pan (or the barbecue) to medium-high heat. Seal the steak on each side for 1 minute, reduce the heat to medium, and continue to cook to your liking. The time for cooking will depend on the thickness of your steak. One tip for cooking the steak, is that the fattier cuts will cook more quickly once the fat heats up – this is why a scotch fillet may take 10 minutes to get to medium, but only a couple more minutes to become well done. Use a meat thermometer if you are unsure, but take care not to prick the meat too many times, as you will lose the delicious juices. Wrap the steaks in foil for 5-10 minutes to rest before serving.

Serve the crayfish and sauce on top of your rested steak, with a salad on the side.

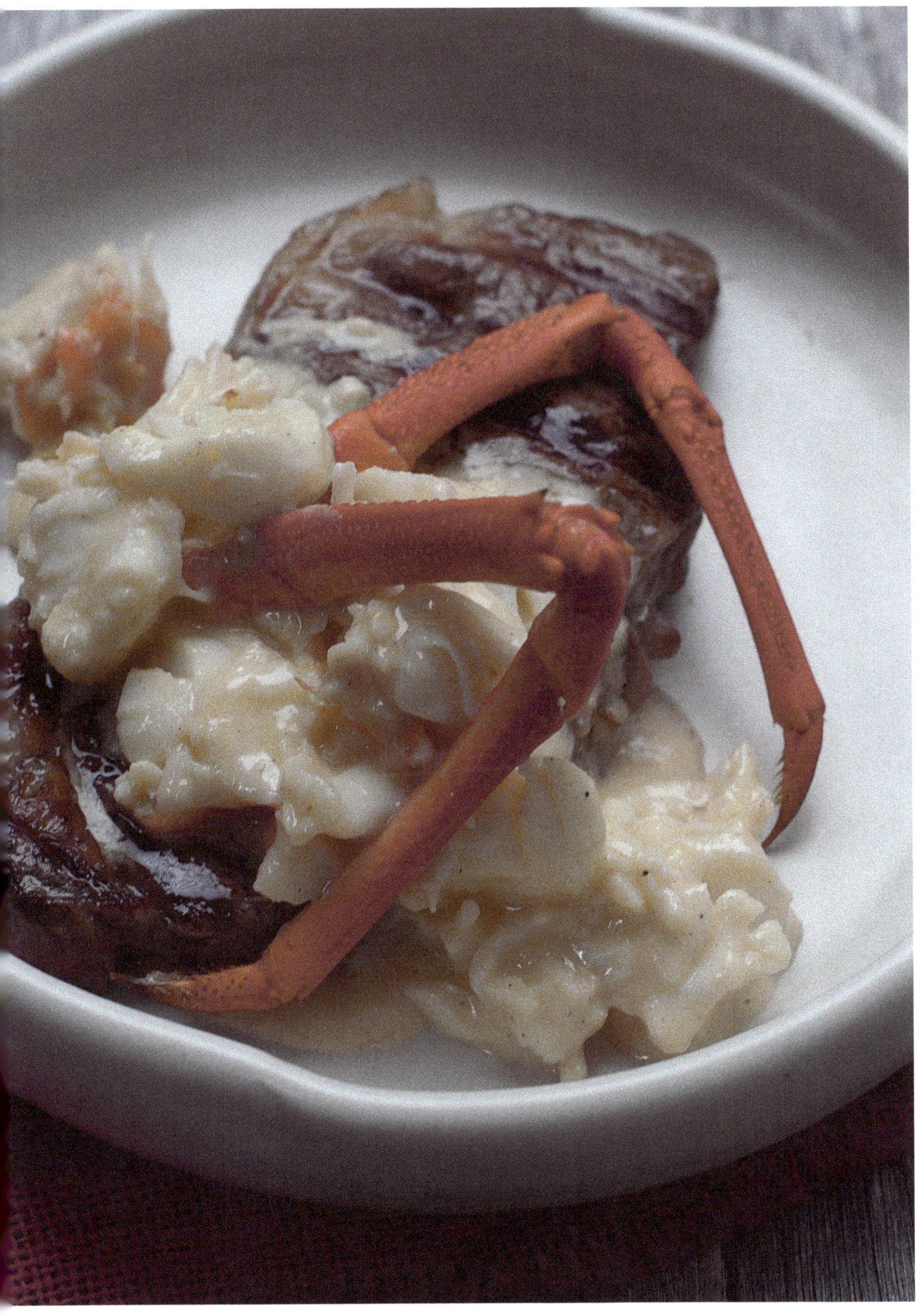

TRACY MARTIN - PETUNA SEAFOODS

Ling Burger with Pickled Onion and Cucumber

SERVES 4

Crumbed Ling makes the best fish burger you could ever dream of! It's also delightful simply steamed or grilled. Pink Ling is a deep sea fish caught year round, making it a very reliable, consistent and versatile fish. Pink Ling is white in flesh with a firm texture that is mild and delicate in flavour. It is suitable for most cooking methods as the fillet maintains its shape.

PICKLED ONION AND CUCUMBER

Spanish onions

2 baby cucumbers

2 teaspoon salt

½ cup white wine vinegar

½ cup caster sugar

TARTARE SAUCE

35 grams gherkins

35 grams capers

1 cup whole egg mayonnaise

lemon juice, to taste

salt and pepper

1 egg

1 cup milk

80 grams rice flour

zest of 1 lemon

2 tablespoons dill

100 grams Panko breadcrumbs

extra virgin olive oil for frying

4 x 120 gram Pink Ling fillets

4 brioche buns

1 baby cos lettuce

To make the pickled onion and cucumber, slice the onion into rings and thinly slice the cumber. Coat in salt and set aside for 30 minutes. Combine the vinegar and sugar in a small saucepan and bring to the boil, remove from the heat and set aside to cool. Rinse the salt off the cucumber and onions, then rest the vegetables in the pickling liquid for 1 hour.

To make the tartare sauce, roughly chop gherkins and capers, mix with the mayonnaise and season with lemon juice, salt and pepper.

To crumb the ling fillets, whisk together the egg and milk to in a bowl. Tip the rice flour into another bowl. Zest the lemon, finely chop the dill and combine with the panko crumbs in a third bowl. Dip each ling fillet into flour, then egg, then press into the breadcrumb mix.

To cook the fish, heat the oil in a frying pan over medium heat, and carefully fry each ling fillet until crisp and golden on each side, this will take 5 -10 minutes depending on the thickness of the fillets.

To assemble the burgers, cut each bun in half, shred the lettuce and add to the bun, add a piece of fish, the picked onions and cucumber, then a generous dollop of tartare sauce. Top with the other bun half and fix with a skewer.

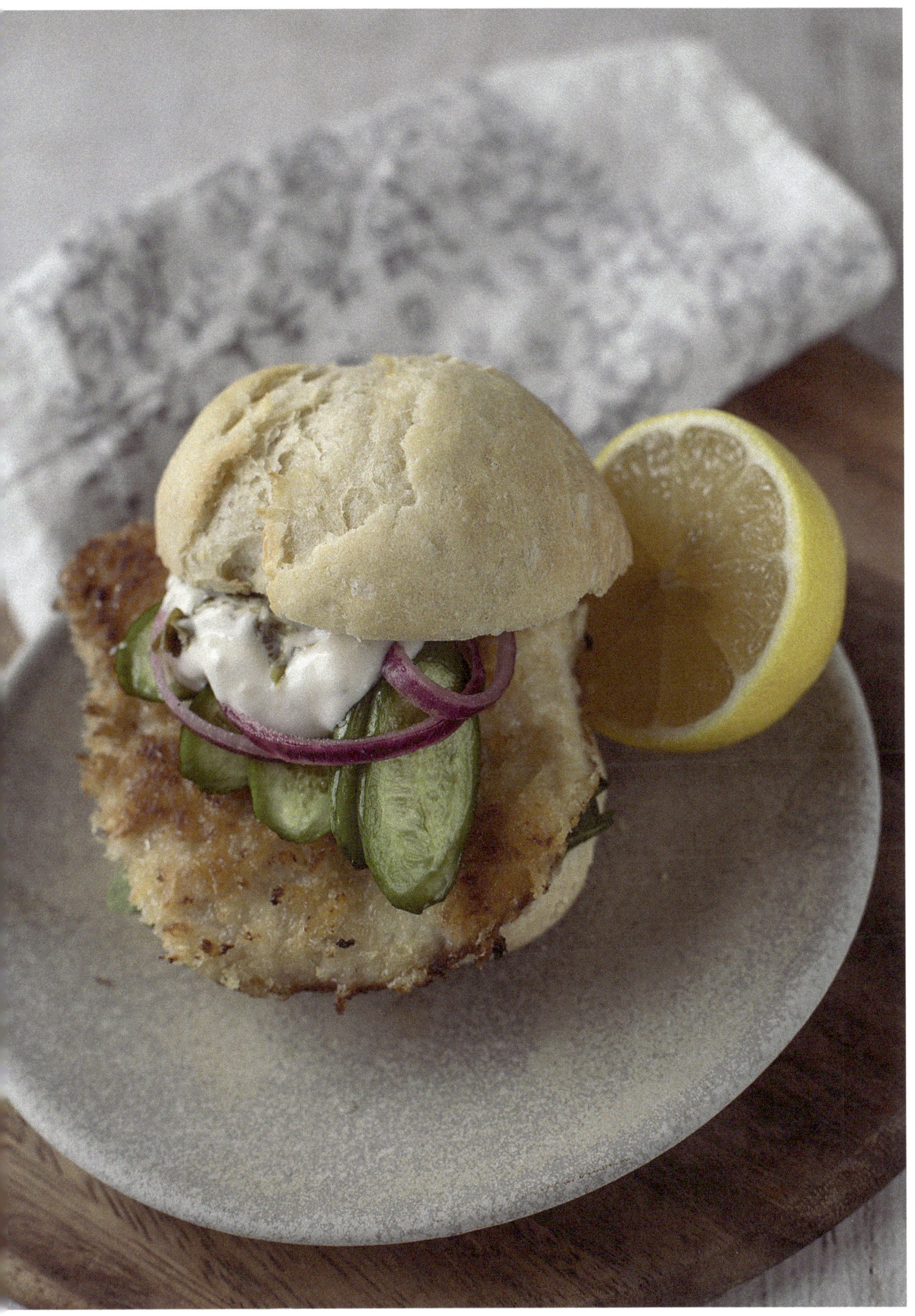

Fennel and Dill Crisp Coated Tuna with Lemon Aioli

SERVES 4

This is a delicious light and crispy way to coat fresh fish. Simply shallow or deep-fry and serve. Blue fin, yellow fin or albacore all work well with this recipe, and you could also use salmon or any other firm, oily, white-fleshed fish.

LEMON AIOLI

2 egg yolks

1 egg

1 tablespoon white vinegar

1 lemon, juice and zest

1 clove garlic salt and pepper

200ml extra virgin olive oil

TUNA

1 egg

½ cup plain flour

½ cup corn flour 1 teaspoon salt

½ teaspoon white pepper

½ teaspoon dried dill

½ teaspoon ground fennel seed

½ teaspoon paprika

4 x 180-200 gram tuna steaks

extra virgin olive oil for deep or shallow frying

To make the aioli, use a blender or food processor to combine the egg yolks, whole egg, vinegar, lemon juice and zest, crushed garlic and a pinch of salt and pepper. While still blending, slowly add the oil in a steady drizzle to create a thick and creamy emulsion.

To cook the tuna, crack the egg into a bowl and whisk lightly with a fork. In a separate bowl, mix the flours with the salt, pepper, dill, fennel and paprika until well combined. Coat each tuna steak in the egg then the flour. Heat a heavy-based pan over a medium high heat, add a dash of oil and cook the tuna steaks for a few minutes on each side, or until crisp and brown.

Tuna is generally served rare in the middle, however if you are cooking a fish that needs to be cooked all the way through, transfer it to a baking dish and put in a 180°C oven to continue cooking, so the outside doesn't burn.

Serve with the aioli and a green salad.

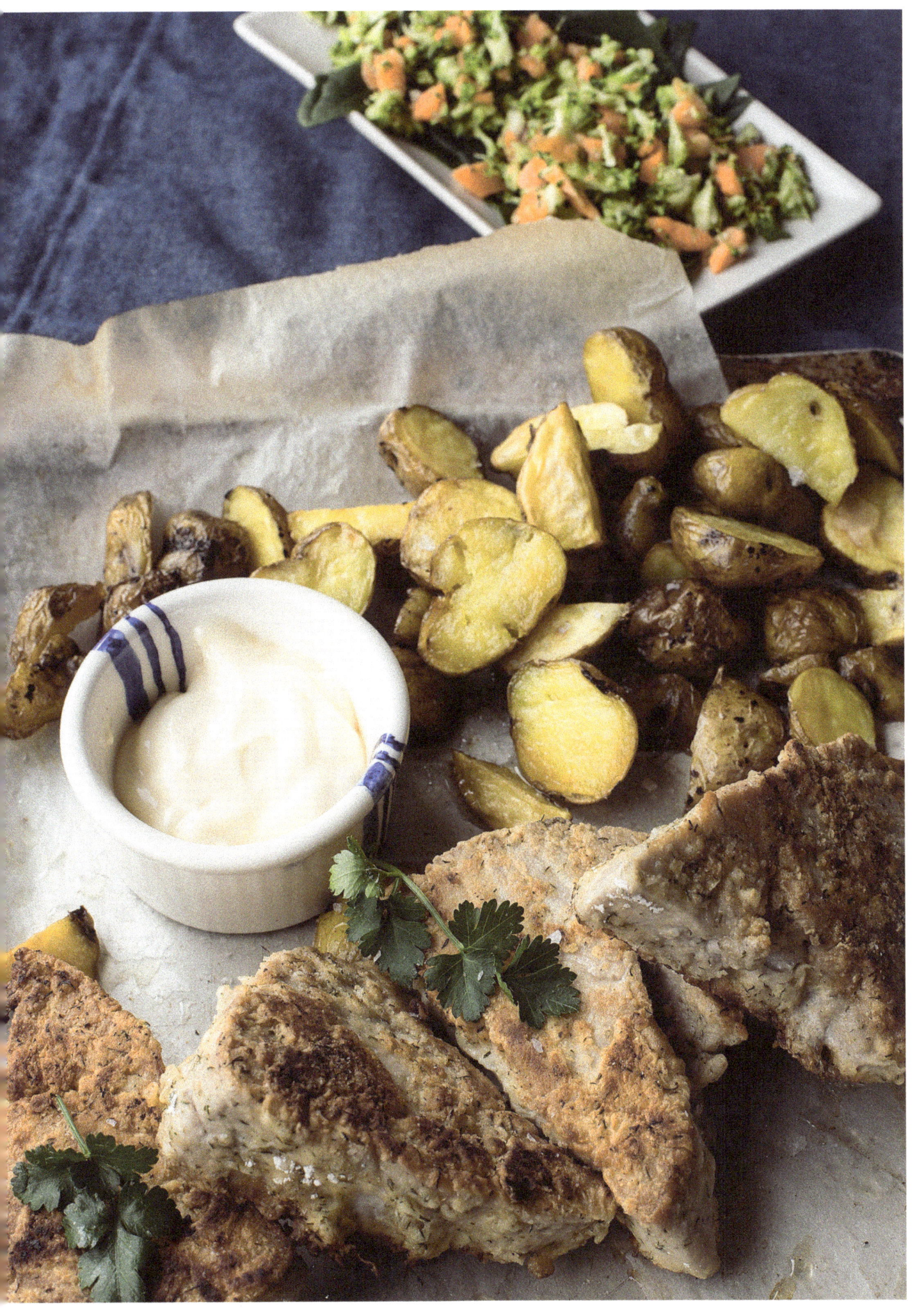

Pan-fried Abalone with Spinach and Feta Salad

SERVES 4 AS AN ENTRÉE

In Tasmania we are still lucky enough to be able to collect an abalone or if you know the right place - with the correct recreation fishing license of course! You will need to prepare this dish quite close to cooking and serving - if you leave the abalone too long the lemon will cook the abalone. If you would rather pre-prepare this dish, simply leave the lemon juice out until just before cooking.

ABALONE

2 abalone

½ large red chilli

1 clove garlic

½ lemon

1 tablespoon oregano

salt and pepper

1 tablespoon butter

2 tablespoons parsley

SALAD

1 capsicum

1 tablespoon extra virgin olive oil

1 clove garlic

½ lemon

2 tomatoes

50 grams Feta cheese

2 cups baby spinach leaves

Start by preparing the abalone. Cut off the black lip by cutting it off and slice across the abalone in horizontal slices, as thin as you can. Bash each slice with a meat mallet to tenderise. Chop the chilli, crush the garlic and mix with the juice and zest of the half of the lemon (keep the other half to use in the dressing) add the chopped oregano and a good pinch of sea salt and pepper.

To make the salad, preheat the oven to 200°C. Brush the capsicum with oil, put in a baking tray and roast for 15 minutes, until the skin blisters. Set aside to cool, then peel the skin off the capsicums.

To make the dressing, crush the garlic and mix with juice from the remaining lemon and finely chopped parsley, then season. Chop the tomatoes and capsicum, crumble the feta cheese, mix well with the spinach leaves and drizzle over the dressing.

To cook the abalone, heat a flat grill or barbecue over high heat, or use a frying pan on the stove. Add the butter and then the abalone and cook for only one minute on each side – the abalone should be golden brown.

Sprinkle with parsley and serve immediately with the salad.

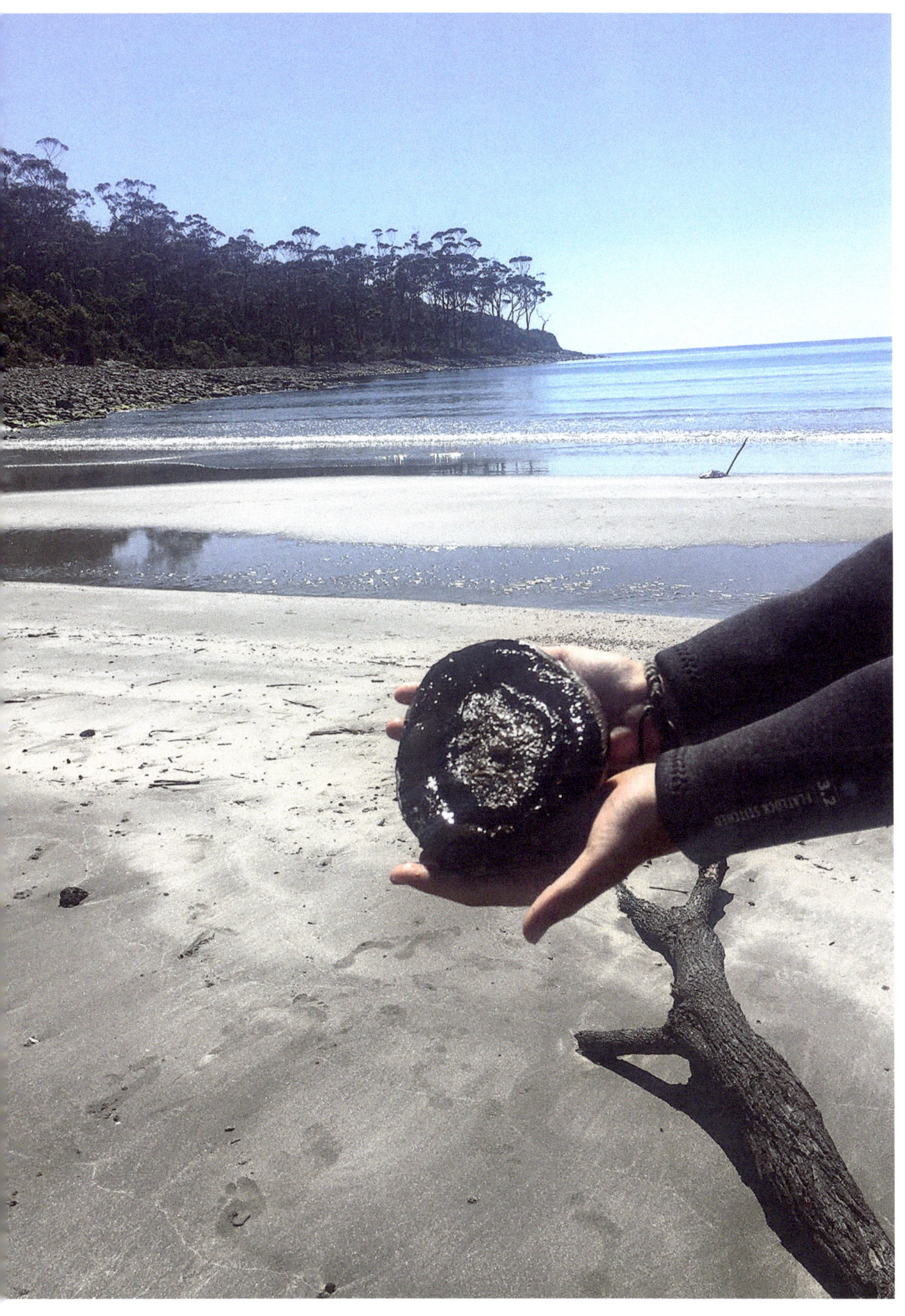

Honey Prawns

SERVES 4

This recipe is for the few lucky recreational fishermen who are able to catch a few prawns for dinner every now and then!

1 clove garlic

1 small onion

1 tablespoon extra virgin olive oil

100ml white wine

200ml cream

1 tablespoon Dijon mustard

1 tablespoon honey

800 grams prawns

To make the sauce, crush the garlic and finely dice the onion. Heat the oil in a heavy-based pan over medium heat and sauté the garlic and onion for 3 minutes, or until softened. Add the wine, bring to a simmer, reduce heat to low and cook until the liquid has reduced by half. Whisk the cream, mustard and honey into the sauce and continue to reduce until the sauce has thickened slightly.

Prepare the prawns by peeling each one and remove the intestine by carefully slicing the back of the prawn and pulling out the dark intestine. Heat the oil in a frying pan over medium heat, add the prawns and cook for 2 minutes each side, or until cooked through. Serve with the hot sauce, rice and salad.

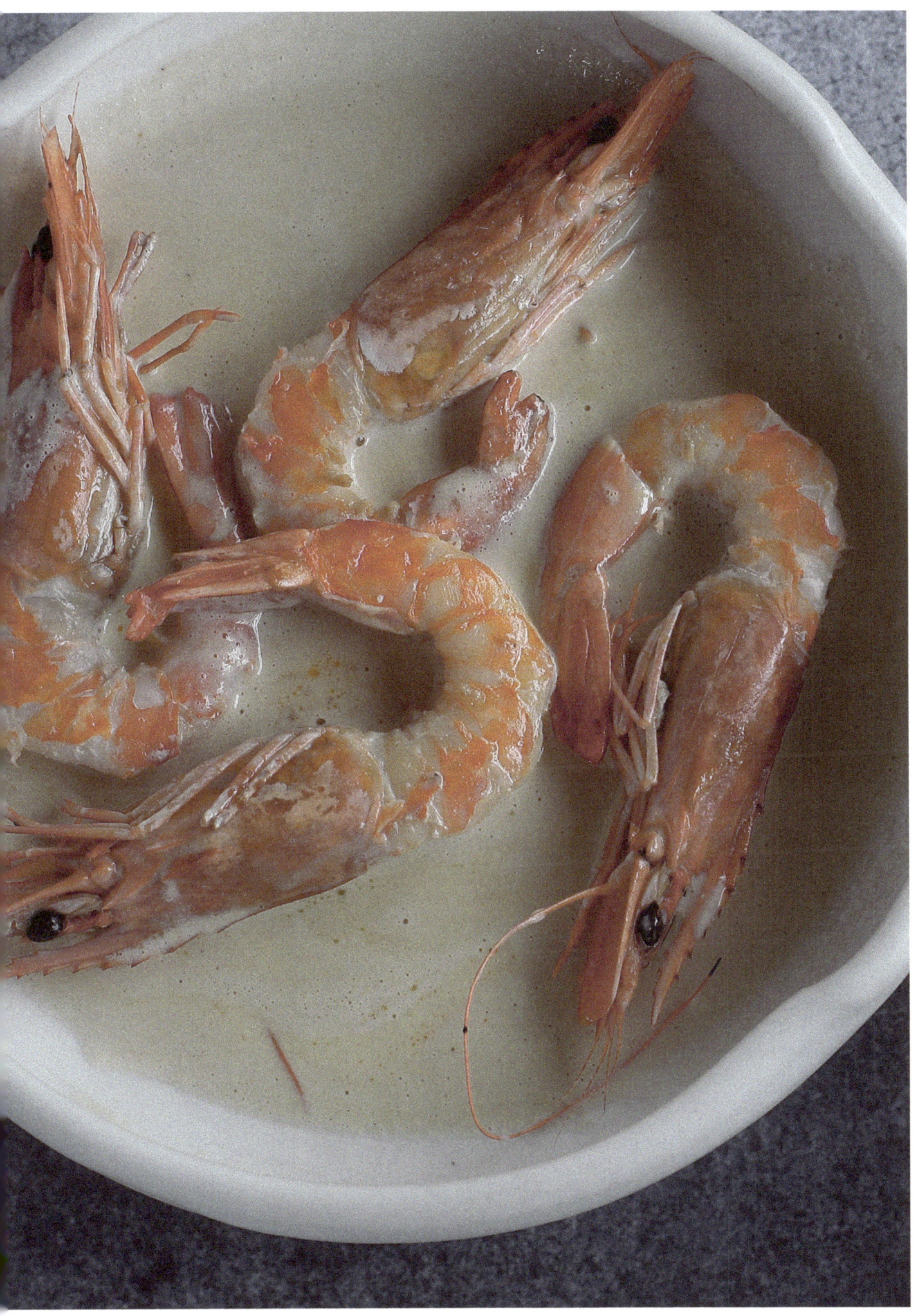

King Fish with Oyster Pâté in Pastry with Lemon Roasted Sweet Potato and Lemon Butter

SERVES 4

This is a lovely dinner party dish that both looks beautiful and is full of flavour. Kingfish is a delicious fish, with a firm white flesh - you could substitute salmon or another white fleshed fish if necessary.

OYSTER PÂTÉ

1 rasher bacon

½ brown onion

½ teaspoon garlic

1 tablespoon extra virgin olive oil

1 dozen smoked oysters

1 teaspoon gelatine powder

15ml brandy

½ tablespoon fresh basil leaves

60ml cream

salt and pepper

KINGFISH PARCELS

1 egg

4 x 200 gram kingfish steaks

4 sheets puff pastry

ROASTED SWEET POTATO

1 medium sweet potato

juice of 1 lemon

2 tablespoons extra virgin olive oil

2 cups spinach leaves

LEMON BUTTER SAUCE

30ml lemon juice

30ml cream

100 grams butter

salt and pepper

To make the oyster pâté, dice the bacon and onion and finely chop the garlic. Heat the oil in a frying pan over medium heat, add the bacon, onion and garlic and fry for 5 minutes, or until the onion is softened and the bacon is cooked. Dissolve the gelatine in a little boiling water and set aside. Add the smoked oysters, brandy, basil and cream to the pan, season with salt and pepper, bring to the boil and add the gelatine mixture. Transfer to a food processor and puree until very smooth, scoop into a bowl and refrigerate until set.

To prepare the kingfish, preheat the oven to 180°C. Make an egg wash by cracking the egg into a small bowl and whisking with a fork. Place each kingfish steak into the middle of a piece of pastry and top the fish with a portion of pâté. Brush the edges of the pastry with egg wash, and fold the corners of the pastry sheet into the middle of the fish, avoiding any overly thick layers of pastry. Place the parcels on a baking tray lined with baking paper and bake for 20 minutes.

Dice the sweet potato into 2-3cm cubes and drizzle with extra virgin olive oil and lemon juice. Bake in the oven for 20 minutes, or until the sweet potatoes are tender and golden.

Make the lemon butter sauce while the potatoes and fish are roasting. Cut the butter into small cubes. Using a small saucepan, bring the lemon and cream to the boil over medium heat, remove from the heat and whisk in the butter. Season to taste with salt and pepper.

To serve, toss the sweet potato with the spinach leaves and serve immediately with the kingfish parcels and lemon butter sauce.

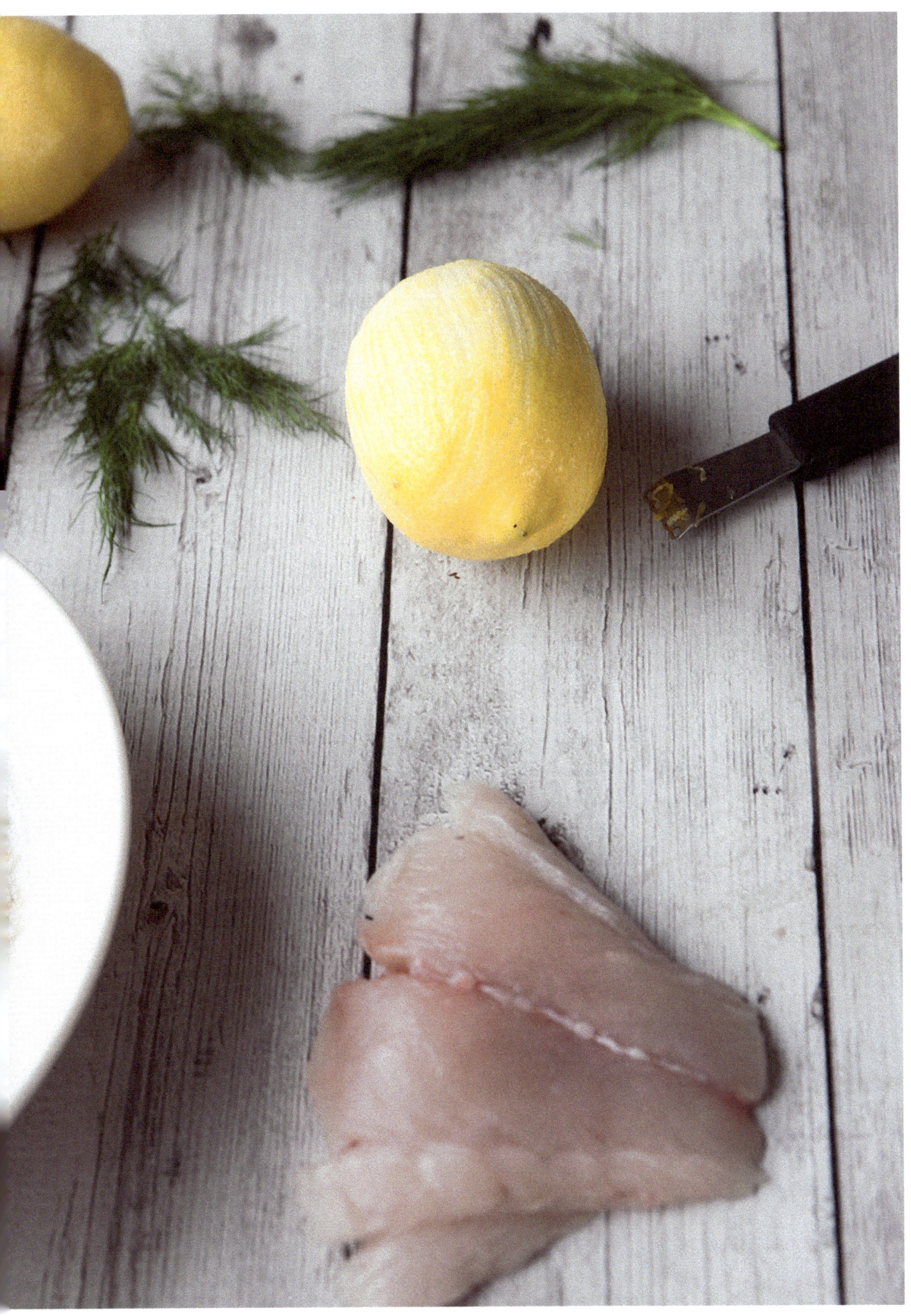

Pickled Octopus with a Greek Salad

MAKES PLENTY

Pickled octopus can be stored in oil for a few weeks and is lovely served with salads, antipasto or as a meal on its own. This is a pickling method that I learnt when I worked in a Greek restaurant – it's a tried and true method that I use all the time!

PICKLED OCTOPUS

1 onion

1 teaspoon garlic

1 large chilli

1 teaspoon oregano

1 kilogram octopus, cleaned and cut into 10cm pieces

½ teaspoon salt

½ teaspoon pepper 1 lemon

1 litre extra virgin olive oil

SALAD DRESSING

1 tablespoon oregano

1 clove garlic

100ml extra virgin olive oil

50ml red wine vinegar

salt and pepper

GREEK SALAD

2 tomatoes

1 medium cucumber

1 red onion

100 grams Feta cheese

100 grams olives

To pickle the octopus, finely chop the onion, garlic, chilli and oregano. Heat the oil in a heavy-based saucepan over medium heat and sauté the onion, garlic, chilli and oregano for a few minutes, or until the onions have softened. Add the octopus pieces and fry until all of the surfaces are sealed. Add the lemon, season with salt and pepper, reduce the heat to low and cook gently for 5 minutes, or until a lot of the liquid has come out of the octopus. Top with enough oil to completely cover the octopus, and cook over low heat for 40 minutes, simmering gently.

Cut a piece of octopus to test if it is cooked – it should be soft, opaque and cooked through. Remove the saucepan from the heat, cover with a lid and set aside to tenderise and cool for at least 3 hours, then refrigerate.

To make the salad dressing, chop the oregano, crush the garlic and mix with the oil, vinegar, salt and pepper. Slice the tomatoes, cucumber and onion, crumble the Feta and combine with the olives.

To serve, assemble the salad and octopus on a plate and drizzle over the dressing.

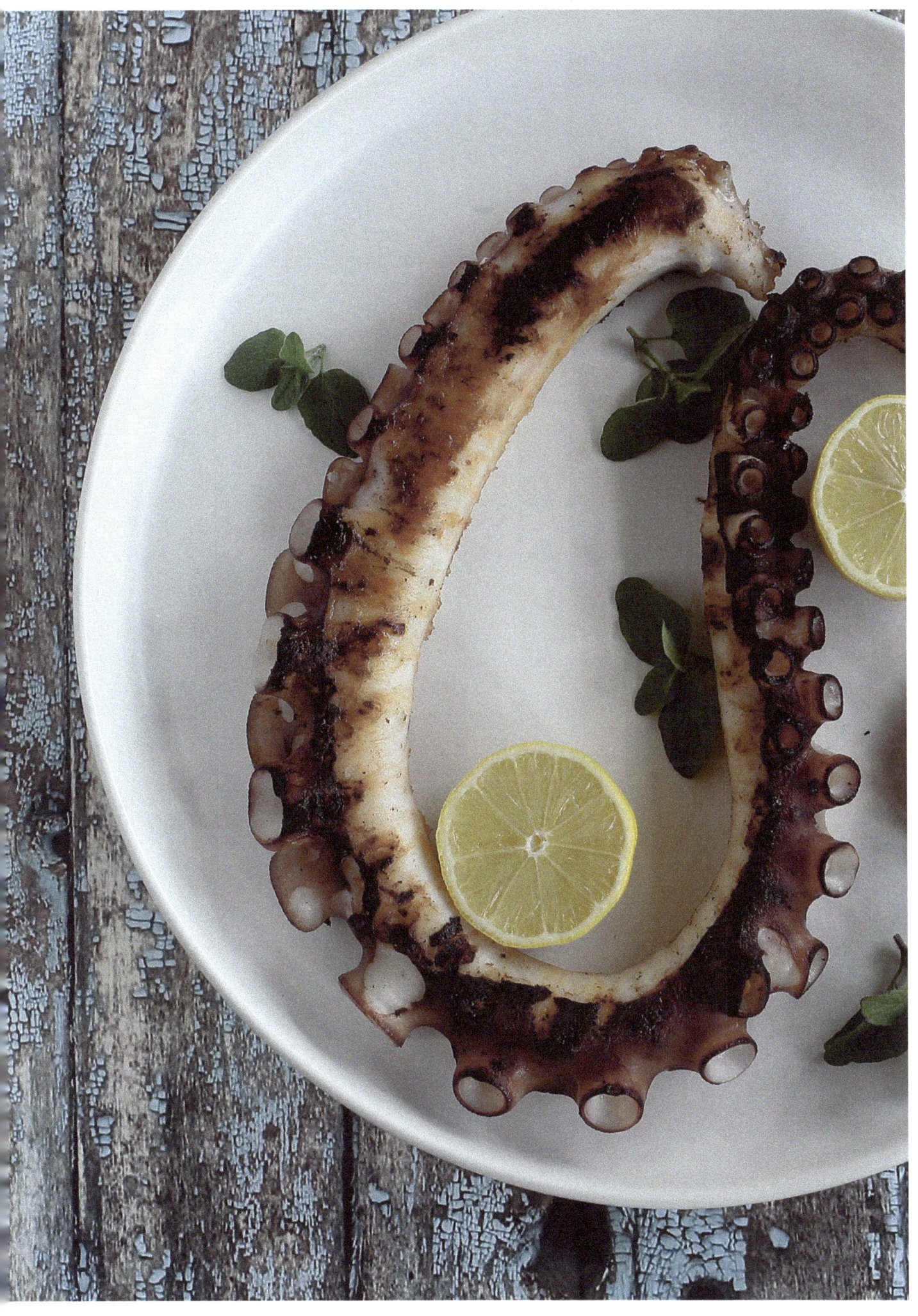

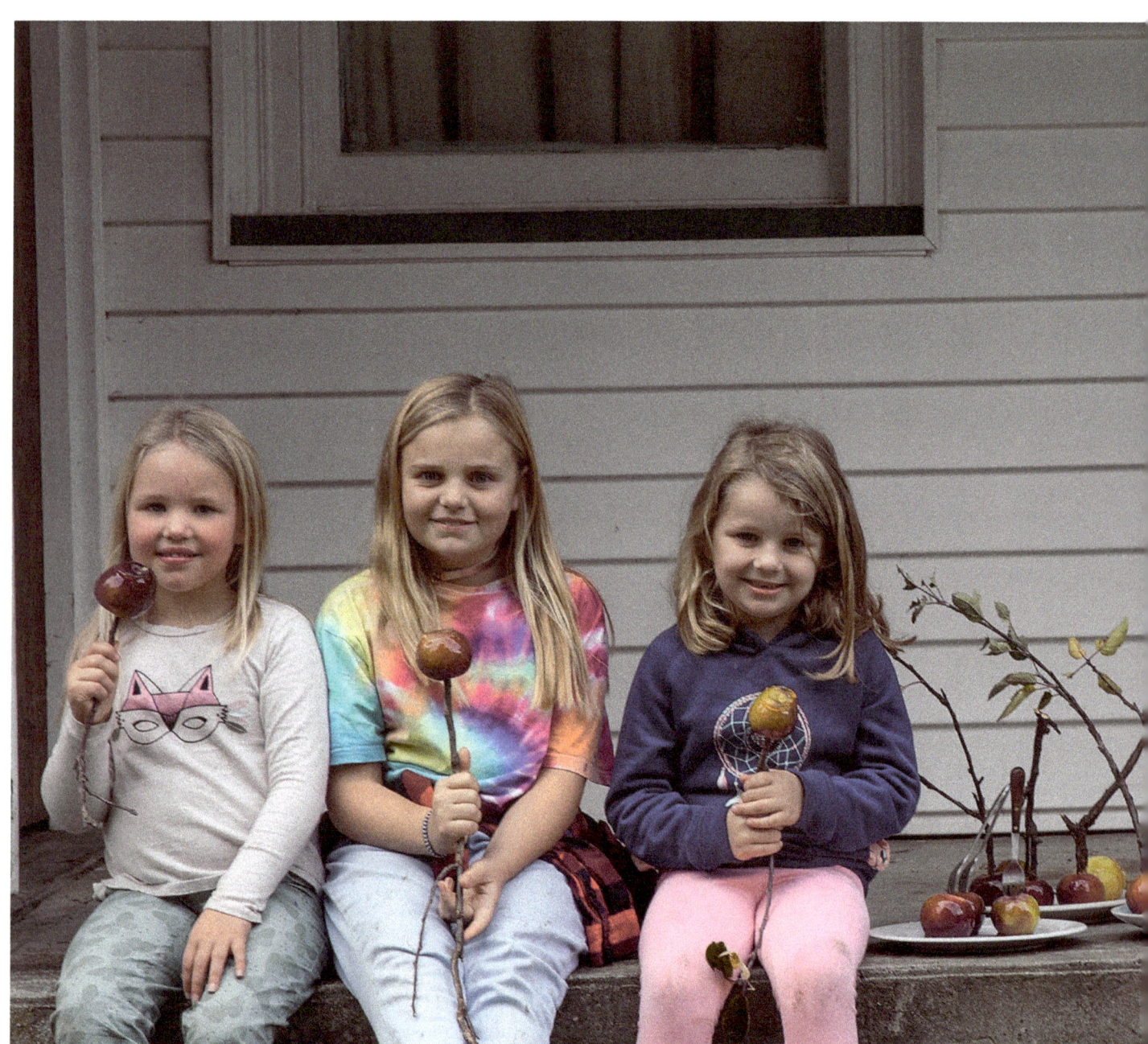

From the Orchard

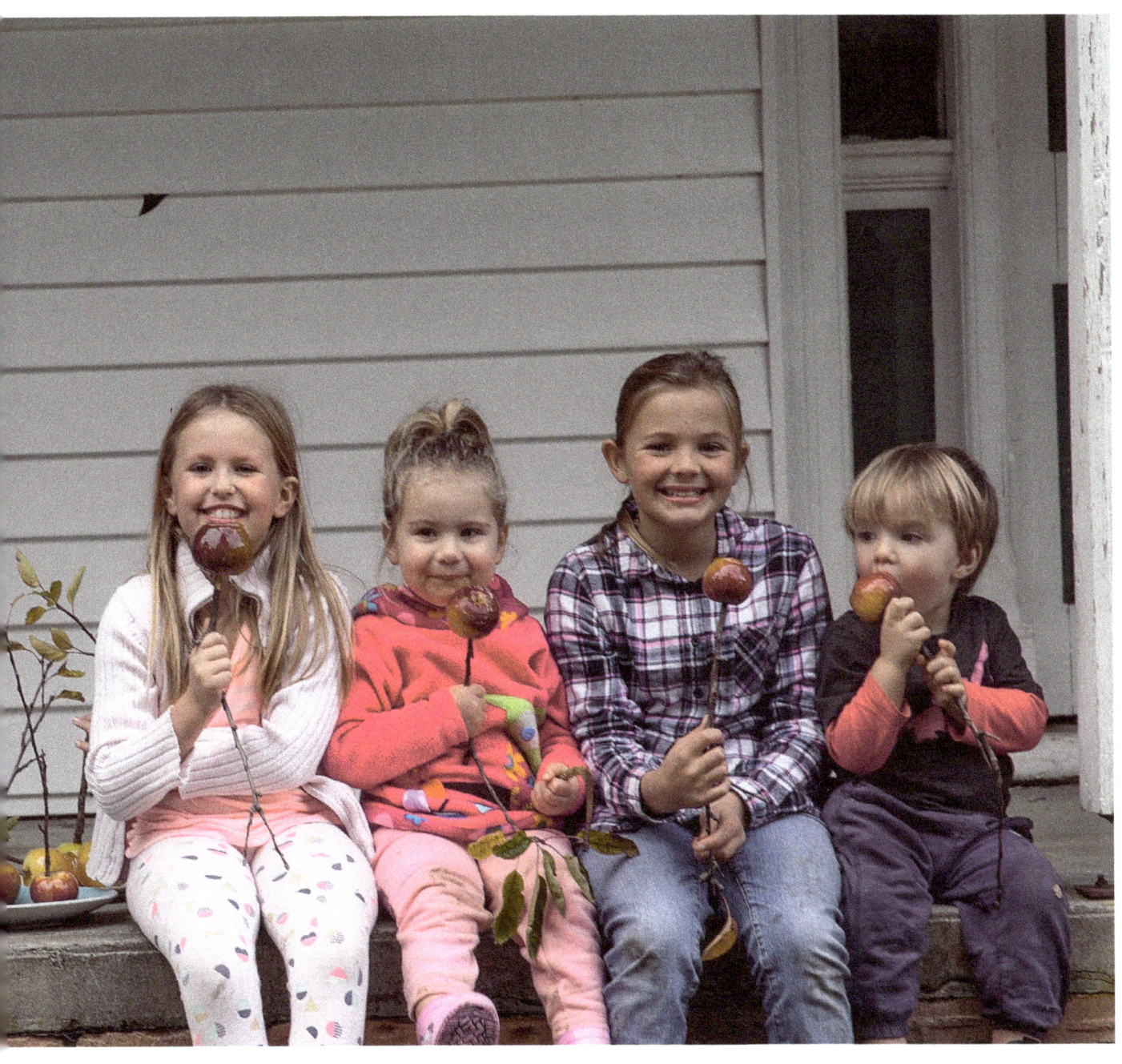

Homemade Toffee Apples

SERVES 12

This is a classic recipe you need to make at least once a year with your kids, it's so much fun! It's also well worth a drive in the Tasmanian countryside in the autumn, just to buy crisp, new seasons apples from a roadside stall.

1 cups sugar

1 teaspoon vinegar

¼ cup water

12 wooden sticks

12 apples

To make the toffee, pour the sugar, vinegar and water into a heavy-based saucepan. Bring the mixture to a simmer over low heat – do not stir and keep the temperature at the lowest heat possible. The mixture will take 10 -15 minutes to start to caramelize and turn a golden brown – keep a careful eye on it as it turns very quickly!

While you are waiting for the toffee to cook, push the sticks firmly into the base of the apples. When the toffee is ready, dip the apples into the hot toffee, and swirl to coat. Be very careful not to touch the toffee, it will be very hot and will burn your fingers! Set aside to cool and set.

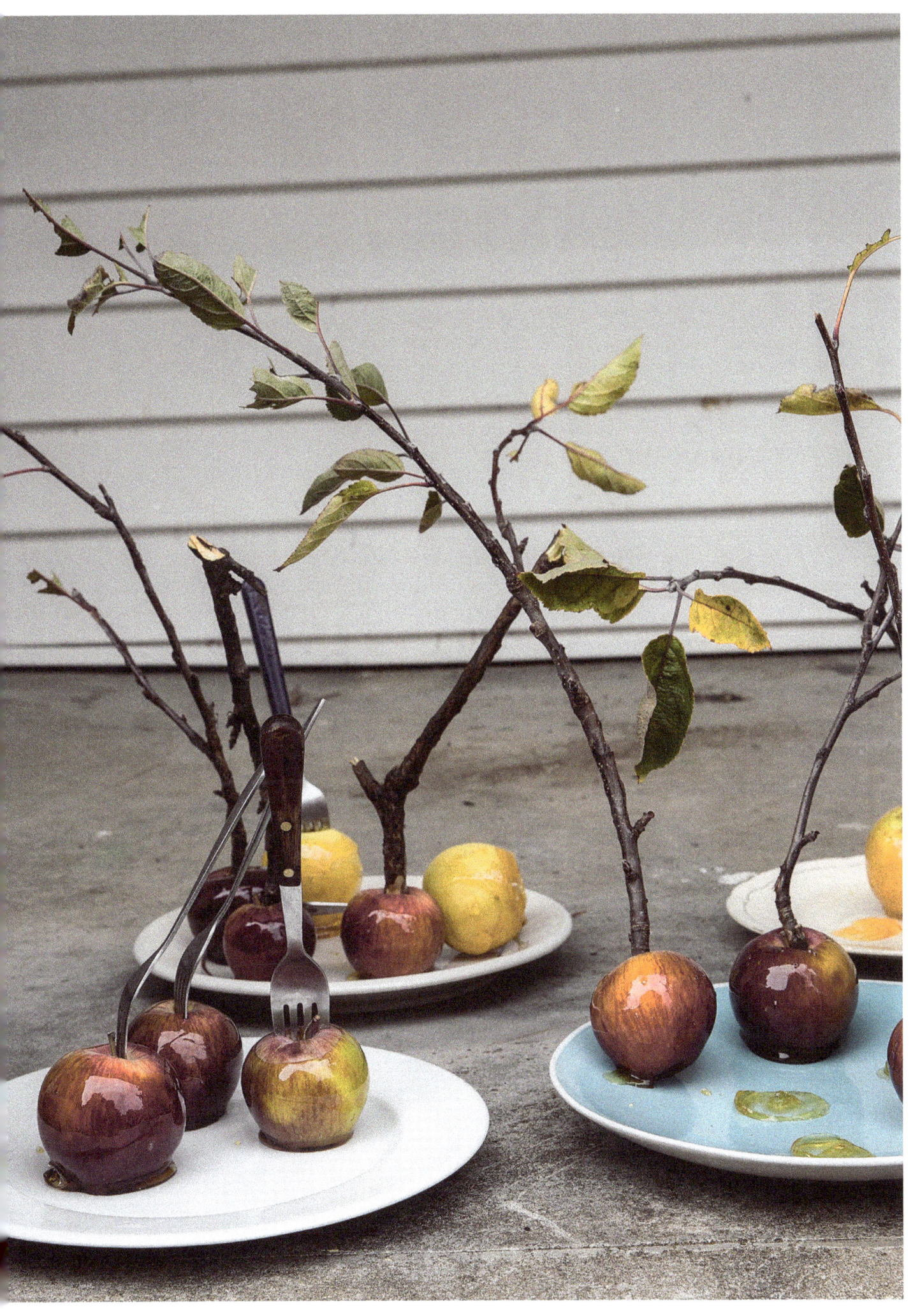

Apple and Blackberry Pie

SERVES 8

Apples are an iconic Tasmanian fruit with the first apple tree planted in the state by Captain Bligh in the 1700s. Since then, apple production has been a vital industry for the state and today most apples in Tasmania are grown in the Huon region with other apple growers in the north of the state such as in Spreyton, where the delicious Spreyton Cider is made. This simple apple pie recipe is also suitable for any stonefruit, once you have tried this easy and light pastry you will make it all the time! Apple and blackberries are a beautiful combination in summer – simply serve with vanilla ice cream and fresh Tasmanian cream.

PASTRY

2 cups self raising flour

¼ cup icing sugar

125 grams butter

½ cup milk

1 egg white

1 tablespoon caster sugar

FILLING

4 apples

1 punnet blackberries

1 tablespoon cornflour

Preheat the oven to 180°C.

Use a food processor to make the pastry. Add the flour, icing sugar and cubed butter to the food processor and pulse until the mixture resembles fine crumbs. Add the milk, a little at a time, and continue to blend until the pastry comes together in a ball. Using 2/3 of the dough, roll the pastry out onto a floured bench to cover the base and sides of a 20cm pie dish. Roll out the remaining pastry for the lid of the pie. Leave the pastry lid on the bench to rest for 20 minutes while you make the filling.

To make the filling, peel, core and dice the apples into 1cm cubes. Tip into a heavy-based saucepan with 1 tablespoon of cold water, place over medium heat and cook for 5-10 minutes, or until the apple is cooked through yet still firm enough to hold its shape. Set aside to cool.

Toss the berries in cornflour, stir into the apple mixture and tip into the pastry-covered pie dish. Lightly whisk the egg white in a small bowl, and brush the egg white around the top edge of the pastry base. Carefully lay the pastry lid on top of the pie and crimp the edges of the pastry together with a fork to seal. Sprinkle with caster sugar. Cut a small hole in the top of the pie to let the steam escape, and bake in the oven for 25 minutes, or until the pastry is golden brown.

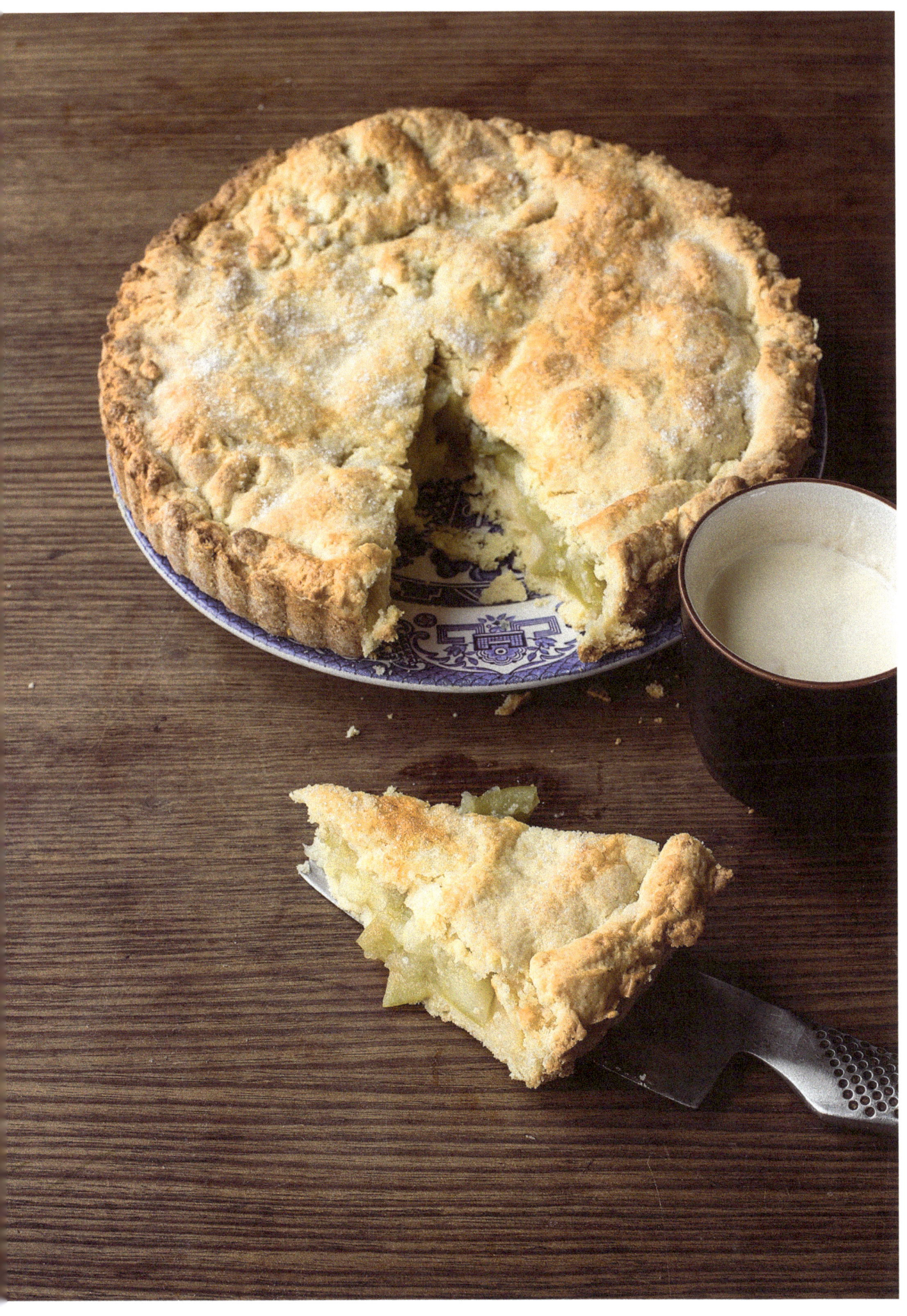

Preserved Lemons

MAKES 4 JARS

Preserved lemons are a staple in Middle Eastern cooking and you can add thin slivers to tartare sauce, homemade hummus or summer salads. A jar will last for a long time and they make lovely gifts.

- 12 lemons
- 2 cups salt
- 4 bay leaves
- 12 cloves
- 8 peppercorns
- 2 cinnamon sticks
- 4 x 290ml clean sterilized jars with lids

Cut each lemon into 8 wedges. Mix the wedges with one cup of the salt and leave to stand for 15 minutes.

Fill the jars with lemon wedges – pushing and squeezing them into the jars with the skin side of the wedge facing out.

While adding the lemons, distribute the bay leaves, cloves, peppercorns and pieces of cinnamon stick throughout the jars. Top the jars with the remaining salt and screw the lids on tightly.

Leave the jars for at least one month before using and refrigerate once opened.

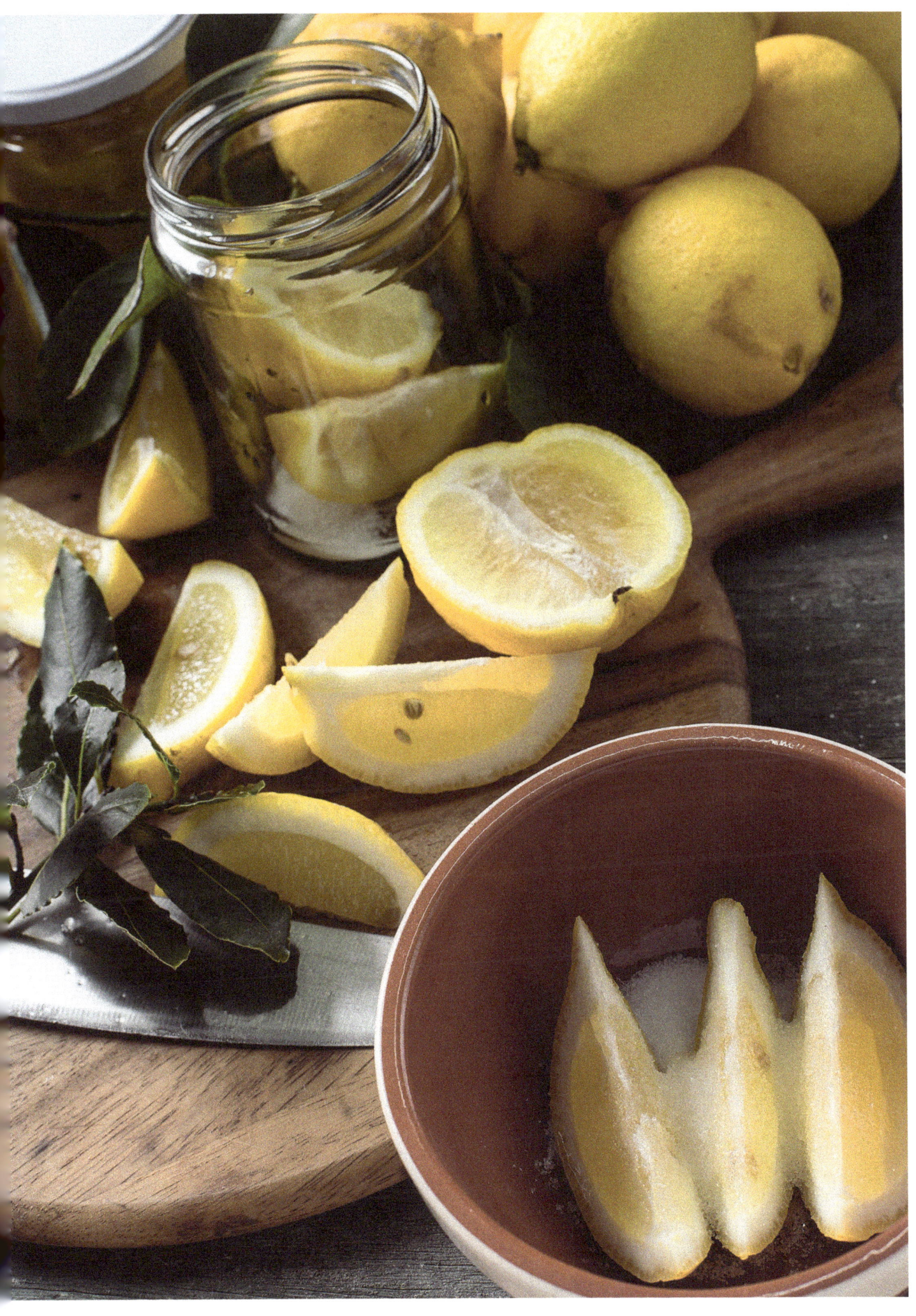

Lemon, Carrot and Polenta Cake With Lemon Syrup (Gluten Free)

SERVES 8

This surprisingly soft and tender-crumbed cake is very easy to make.

- 150 grams almonds
- 2 carrots
- 4 lemons
- 150 grams butter
- 160 grams polenta
- 1 ½ teaspoon baking powder
- 3 eggs
- 60 grams honey
- 150 grams sugar

Preheat the oven to 180°C. Grease and line a 20cm cake tin.

To make the cake, use a food processor to blend the almonds to a fine powder. Grate the carrots, zest and the juice the lemons, setting the juice aside to use in the syrup later.

Using a large bowl, combine the almonds, carrot, lemon zest, softened butter, polenta, baking powder, eggs and honey and beat well until incorporated.

Alternatively, use a Thermomix to blend all the ingredients on speed 10 for one minute. Tip into the prepared tin and bake for approximately 25 minutes, or until cooked through.

To make the syrup, combine the lemon juice and sugar in a small saucepan over low heat, and bring to a gentle simmer, cooking for a few minutes or until the sugar is dissolved. Leave to cool before pouring over the cake.

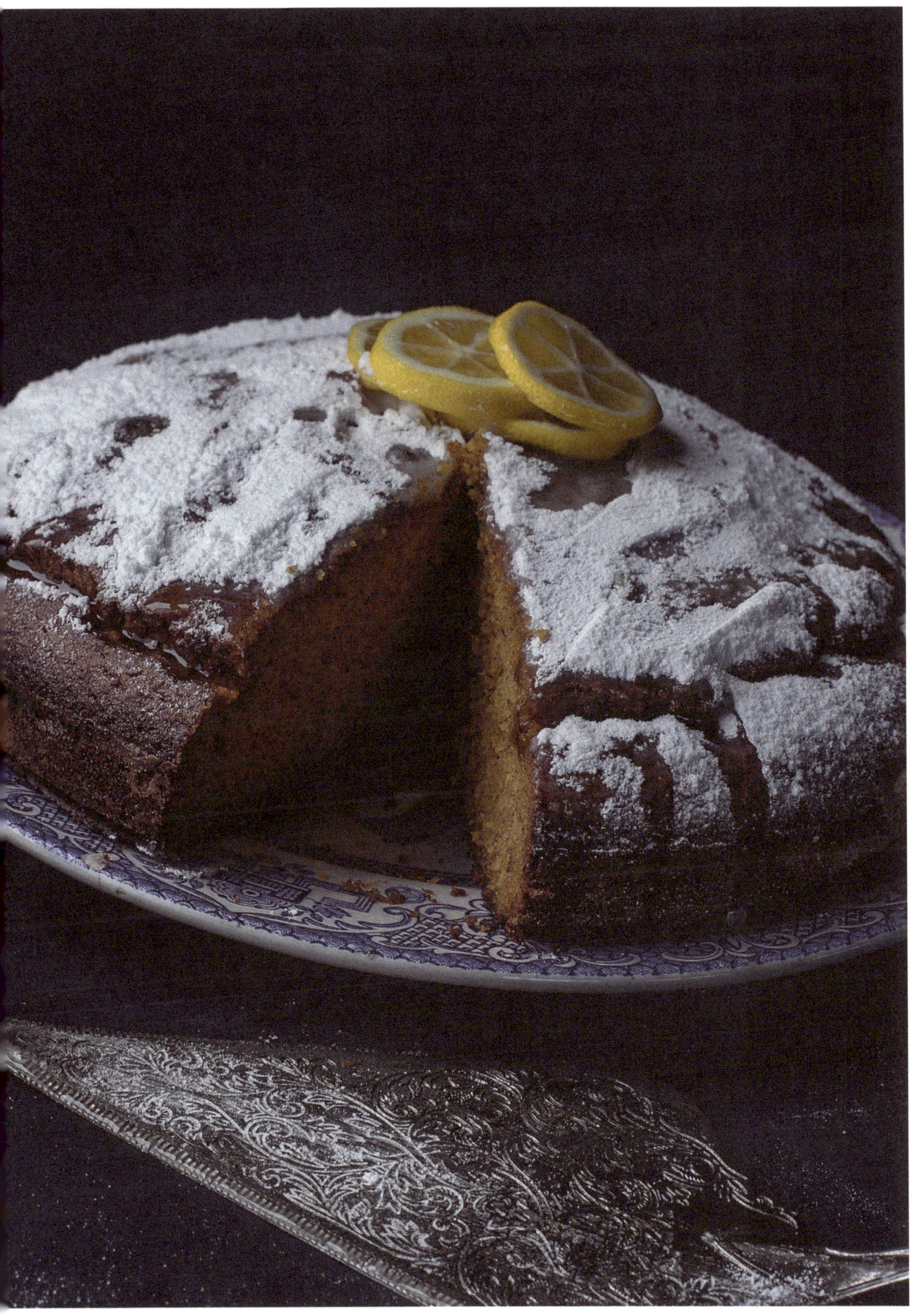

Lemon Tart

SERVES 8, GENEROUSLY

BASE

240 grams plain flour

1 tablespoon sugar

180 grams butter

2 tablespoons water

FILLING

4 medium lemons

6 eggs

100 grams sugar

100ml cream

Preheat the oven to 180°C.

Use a food processor to make the pastry base. Tip the flour and sugar into the processor, add the cubed butter and pulse until the mixture resembles fine breadcrumbs. With the motor running, add the water and blend until the mixture comes together into a firm dough.

Grease a 20cm tart tin and sprinkle with flour. Roll the pastry out on a floured bench and line the base and sides of the tin, then set aside to rest for at least 30 minutes.

To make the filling, zest and juice the lemons, and beat with the eggs, sugar and cream until well combined. Pour into the pastry base and bake for 30 minutes, or until the filling is set.

Remove from the oven and set aside to cool before serving.

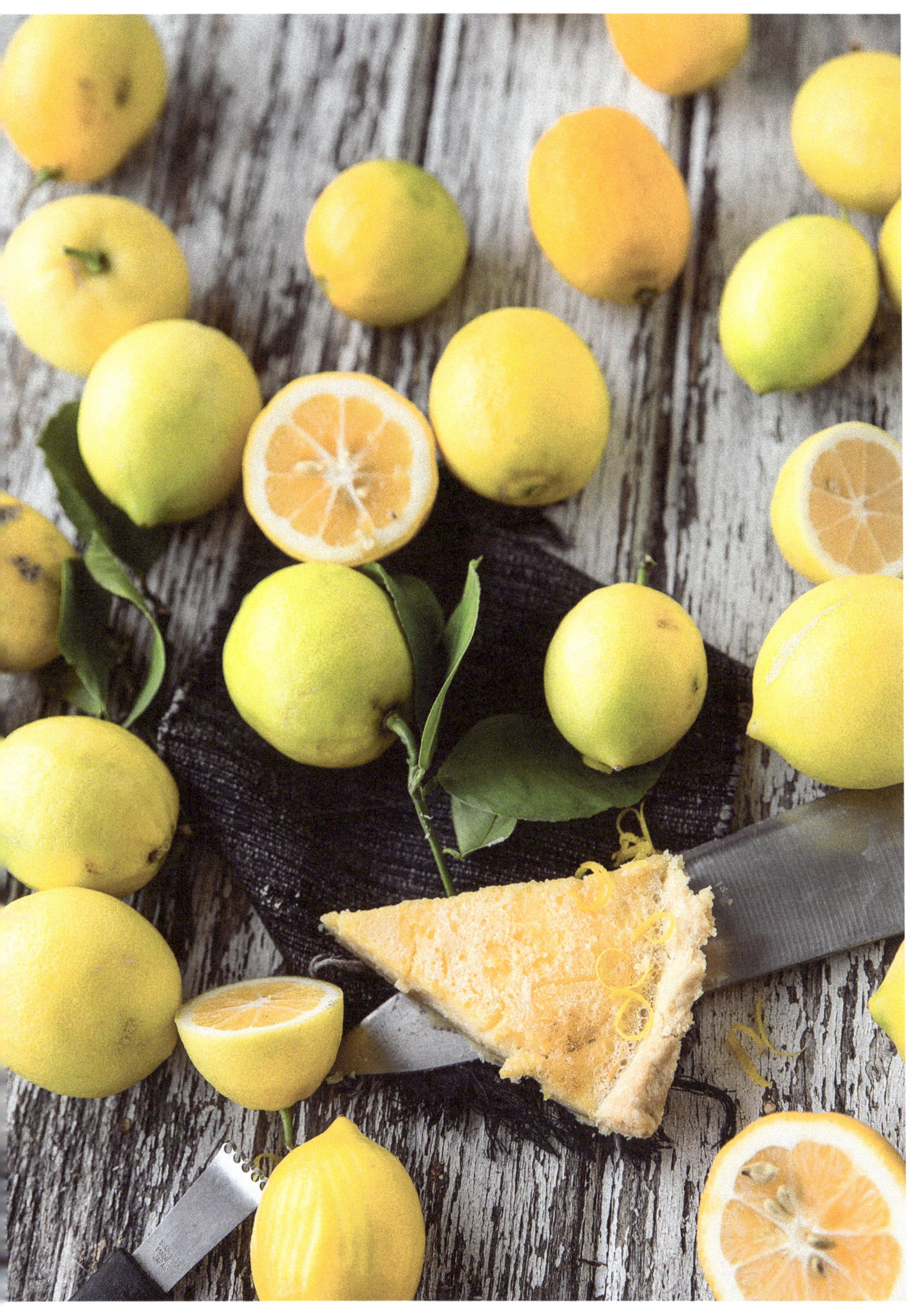

Quince Paste

MAKES A KILO OR 2

This recipe makes plenty of quince paste – enough to share with lucky family and friends and to keep some for yourself too, of course! Not only is it delicious served with cheese, but I always add a tablespoon or two to my gravy or stews as well. The beauty of this recipe is that you can use the whole quince – skins, core and pips and it is such an easy method! You will return to it again and again.

1 kilogram quinces
500ml water
1 kilogram sugar

Chop the whole quinces into 2cm pieces. Tip into a heavy-based pot, add the water, bring to a gentle simmer over medium heat and cook for 30 minutes, or until the fruit is cooked and very soft, stirring occasionally.

Using a stick blender, puree until the mixture is a smooth consistency. Add the sugar, return to a simmer and cook for one hour, or until the mixture thickens and turns a deep, dark, red colour. Stir the mixture regularly to ensure that it doesn't stick to the bottom of the saucepan.

Pour into a tray lined with plastic wrap, set aside to cool and place into the refrigerator to set.

Once set, cut into pieces and wrap in waxed paper. Store in a container in the fridge or freezer until required.

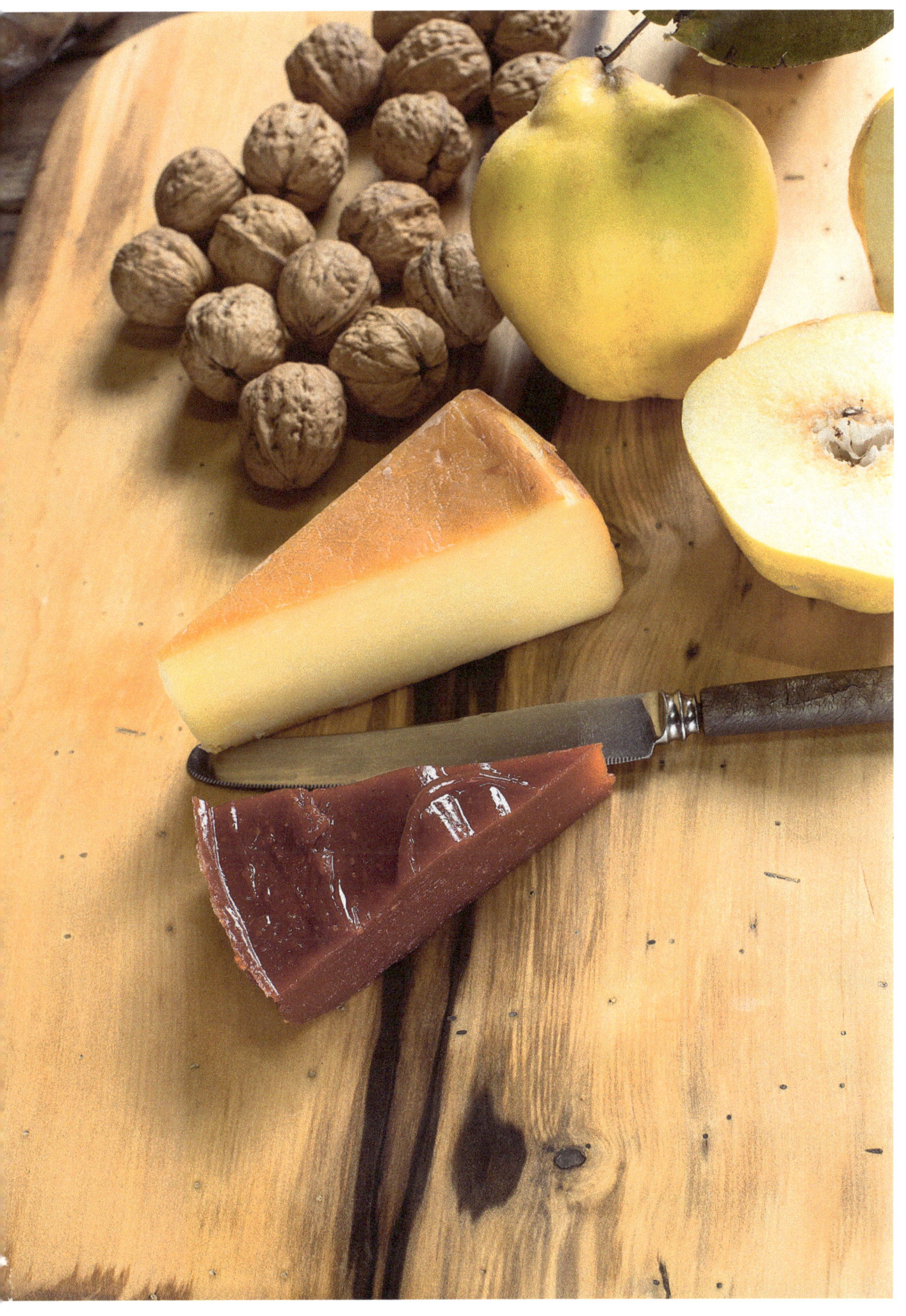

Apple Crumble

SERVES 8

This crumble topping works well with all stewed fruit. If you make a double batch of crumble topping you can freeze the excess and sprinkle on top of seasonal fruit for a super quick and easy dessert.

APPLES

6 large apples

1 tablespoon sugar

CRUMBLE TOPPING

80 grams butter

60 grams rolled oats

120 grams self-raising flour

100 grams brown sugar

Preheat the oven to 180°C.

Peel and core the apples, and dice into 1cm cubes. Tip into a heavy-based saucepan with the sugar and cook over low heat for 10 minutes, or until softened. Tip the apples into a casserole dish.

To make the crumble topping, cut the butter into cubes, combine the oats, flour and sugar in a large bowl. Rub the butter into the flour mixture with your fingers. Mix well and sprinkle over the apples.

Bake in the oven for 20 minutes, or until golden brown and bubbling at the edges. Serve with ice cream or fresh cream.

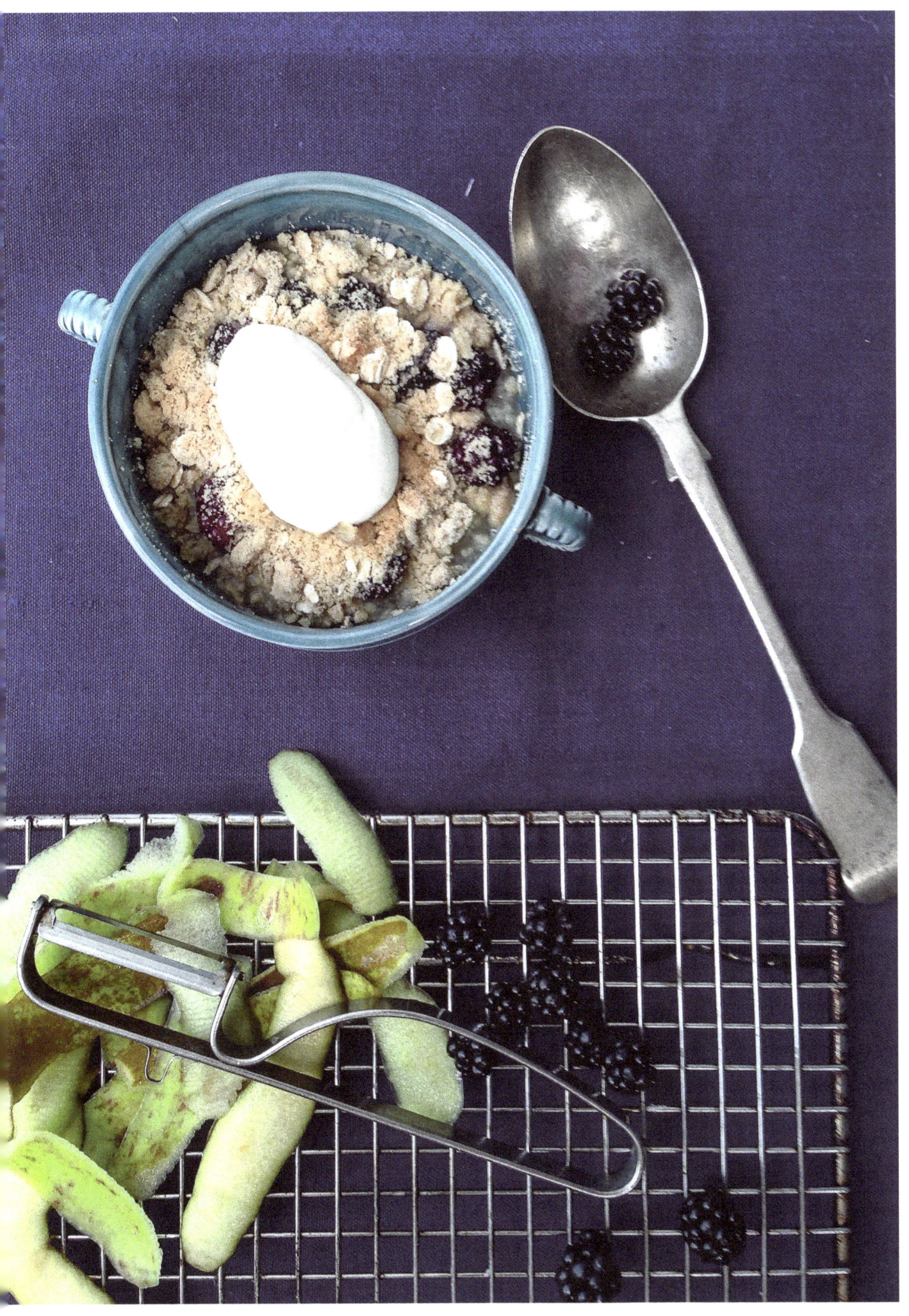

Apple Crumble Slice

SERVES 8

This is a versatile recipe; you could use pears, apricots, nectarines or quinces in place of the apples – just ensure you have around 400 grams of cooked fruit in total (steamed, boiled, sautéed, poached or stewed will all work). You could also mix seasonal fruits together, and add some berries to the mix. If using quinces, they will need to be peeled, cored and quartered. Put them into a large, heavy-based saucepan, cover with water and poach for 30 minutes, or until the quinces are soft and have turned pink – you can add sugar to taste if you wish, but I find that they are sweet enough with the sugar added to the cake base, crumble and ice cream.

6 apples

sugar to taste if necessary

CRUMBLE TOPPING:

100 grams butter

100 grams oats

150 grams self raising flour

100 grams brown sugar

1 teaspoon cinnamon

BASE

200 grams butter

150 grams caster sugar

2 eggs

150 grams plain flour

150 grams self-raising flour

5 grams cinnamon

Preheat the oven to 180°C and line a 20cm cake tin with baking paper.

Peel and core the apples, and dice into 1cm cubes. Tip into a heavy-based saucepan with the sugar and cook over low heat for 10 minutes, or until softened.

To make the crumble topping, cut the butter into cubes, combine the oats, flour, sugar and cinnamon in a large bowl. Rub the butter into the flour mixture with your fingers. Mix well and set aside.

To make the base, cream the softened butter and sugar together until light and creamy. Beat in the eggs and mix until well combined. Fold in the flours and cinnamon, and pour into the cake tin, using a spatula to spread into an even layer. Top with the cooled apple (or other fruit) and then top with the crumble mixture. Bake for 25 minutes, or until cooked through and golden brown on top.

To make the base in the Thermomix, cream the butter and sugar for 15 seconds on speed 5 (scraping the sides if necessary). Add the eggs and mix for 10 seconds on speed 5, add the flours and cinnamon and mix for 10 seconds on speed 5. Proceed with the recipe as above.

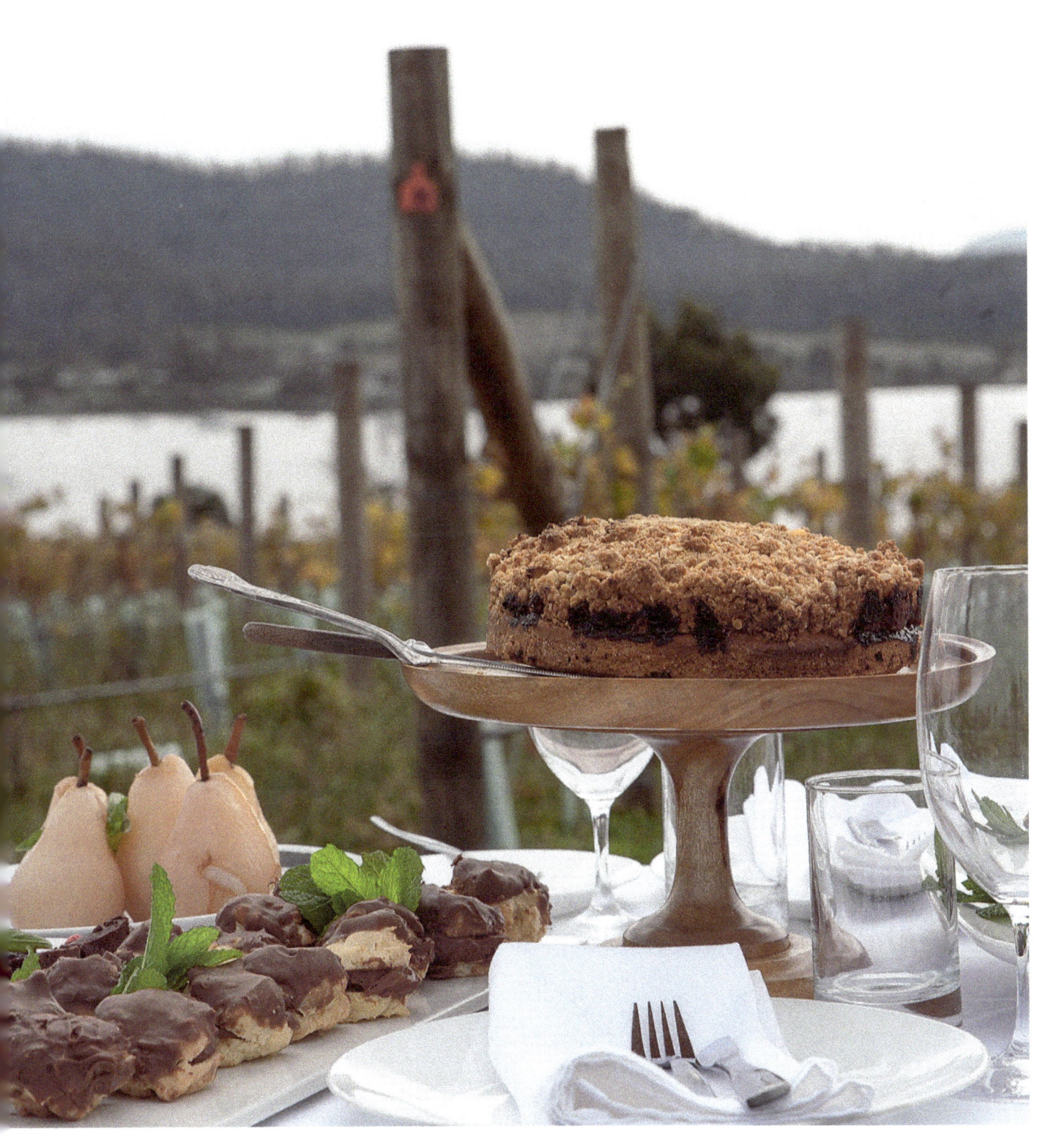

Nashi Pear Tarte Tartin

SERVES 4

These gorgeous little individual-sized tarts work beautifully if you have a set of single serve oven-proof frying pans. Alternatively you can use individual ramekins – just add the sautéed pears to the bottom of the ramekins, top with pastry and bake as directed. To make one large tart, sauté all of the pears and top with a large pastry circle to fit the frying pan.

4 medium nashi pears

1 sheet puff pastry

4 teaspoons butter

4 tablespoons brown sugar

Preheat the oven to 180°C.

Peel, core and thinly slice the nashi pears. Using the frying pan as a guide, cut four circles of pastry from the pastry sheet.

Using a small, individual-sized oven-proof frying pan, melt a teaspoon of butter over low heat and sauté the slices of one pear for two minutes, or until soft.

Add one tablespoon of brown sugar and sauté for one more minute, or until the sugar has dissolved. Arrange the pear slices in the pan and lay a pastry circle on top of the pears.

Gently push the edges of the pastry down the sides of the frying pan. Repeat with the other 3 pans or ramekins. Bake in the oven for 25 minutes, or until the pastry is cooked through and golden brown.

Remove from the oven and carefully turn the tarts out of the frying pans, flipping them over so that the pastry is on the bottom and the pears on the top.

Serve immediately with cream and ice cream.

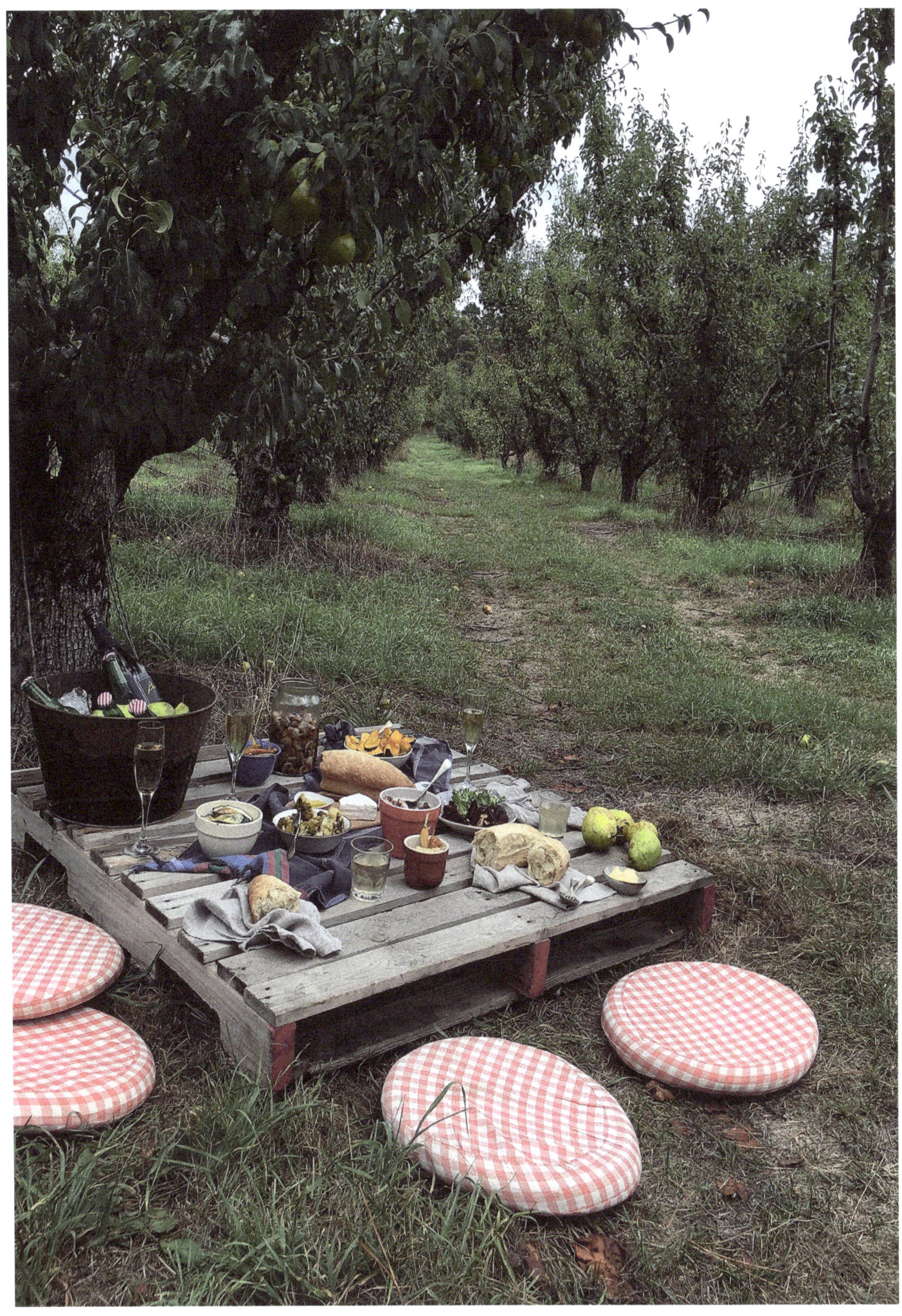

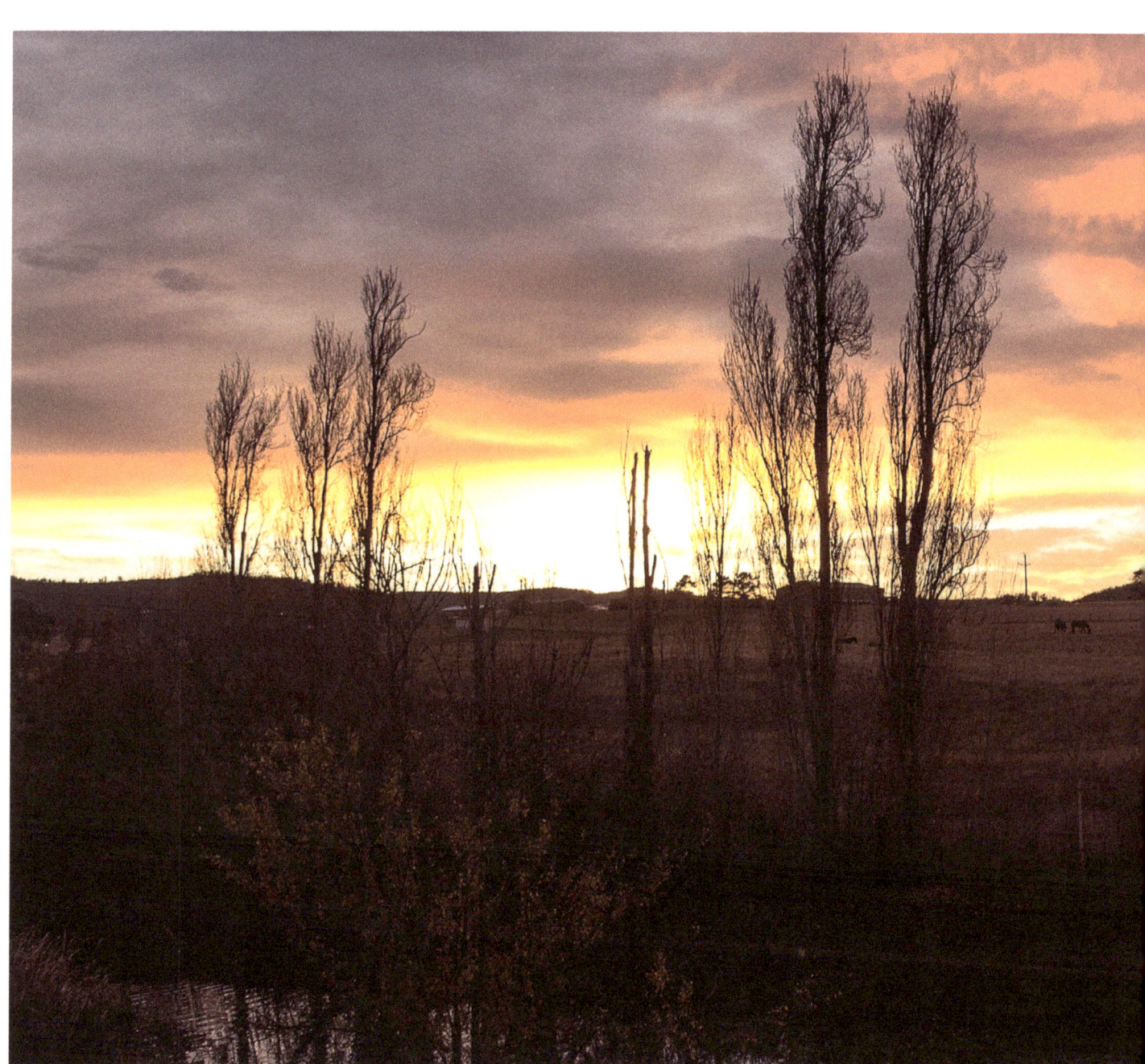

Feathered

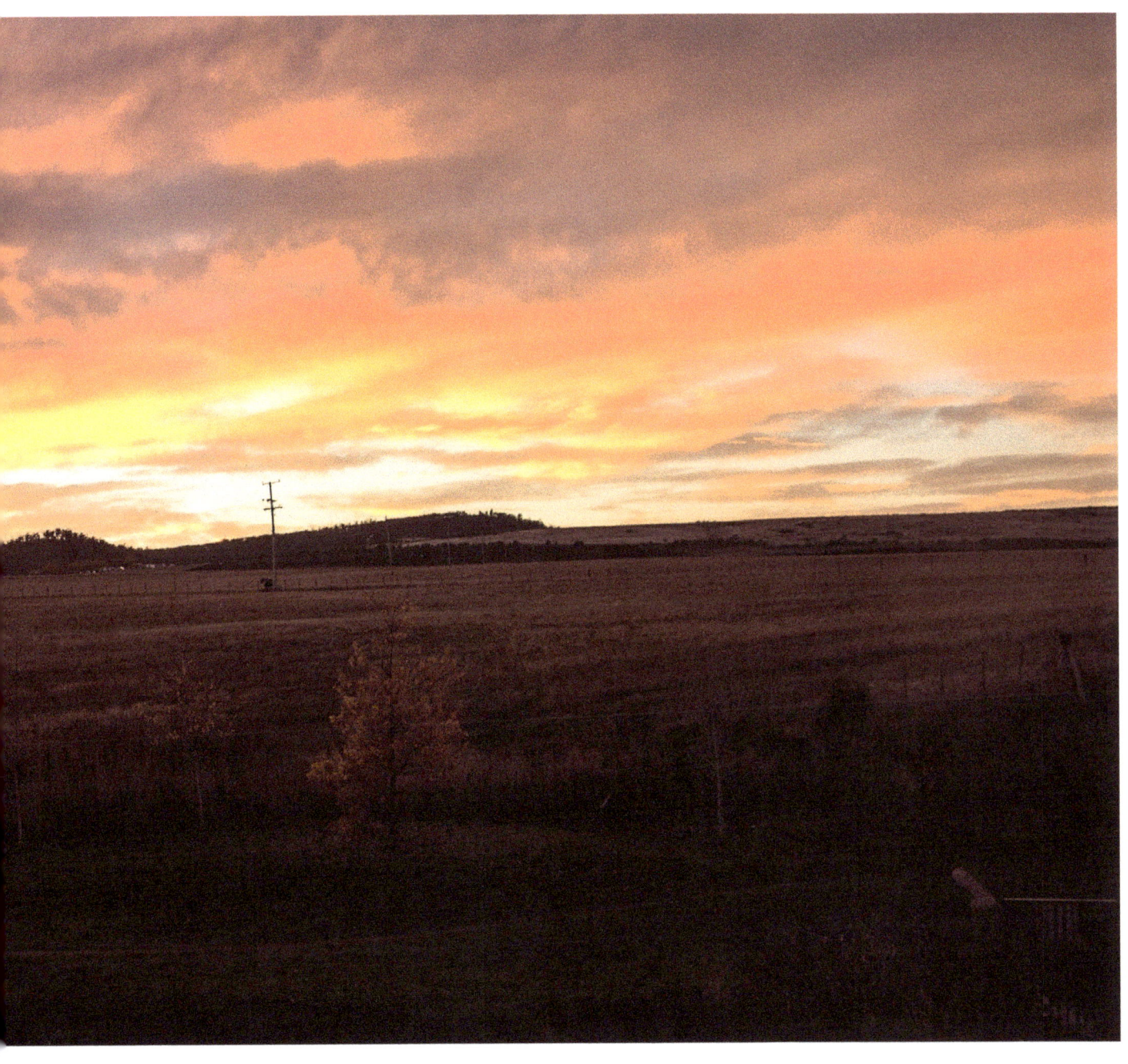

Slow Cooked Duck

SERVES 2-4

This is a very easy way to prepare a duck in the slow cooker. If you want to cook more than one duck, use a deep baking tray, cover well and cook in the oven at 150°C for 3-4 hours. Although not a huge commercial industry in Tasmania you will find ducks on smaller farms, and in the wild. This slow cooked duck is delicious served with veggies or shredded and served over a salad.

2 carrots

1 onion

1 stick celery

1 whole duck

1 teaspoon crushed dry Tasmanian pepper berries

1 tablespoon quince paste

1 tablespoon honey

1 tablespoon seeded mustard

pinch salt

Peel and roughly chop the carrots and onion, roughly chop the celery and tip the vegetables into the bottom of the slow cooker.

With the fatty breast side up, place the duck on top of the vegetables and tuck the neck and wings underneath the bird.

Mix the pepper berries, quince paste, honey and mustard together in a small bowl, and rub into the skin of the bird. Put the lid on the slow cooker and turn on to cook on high for 4-6 hours.

There is a big difference in the time it takes to cook in different brand slow cookers, so just be aware of this, and get to know your own.

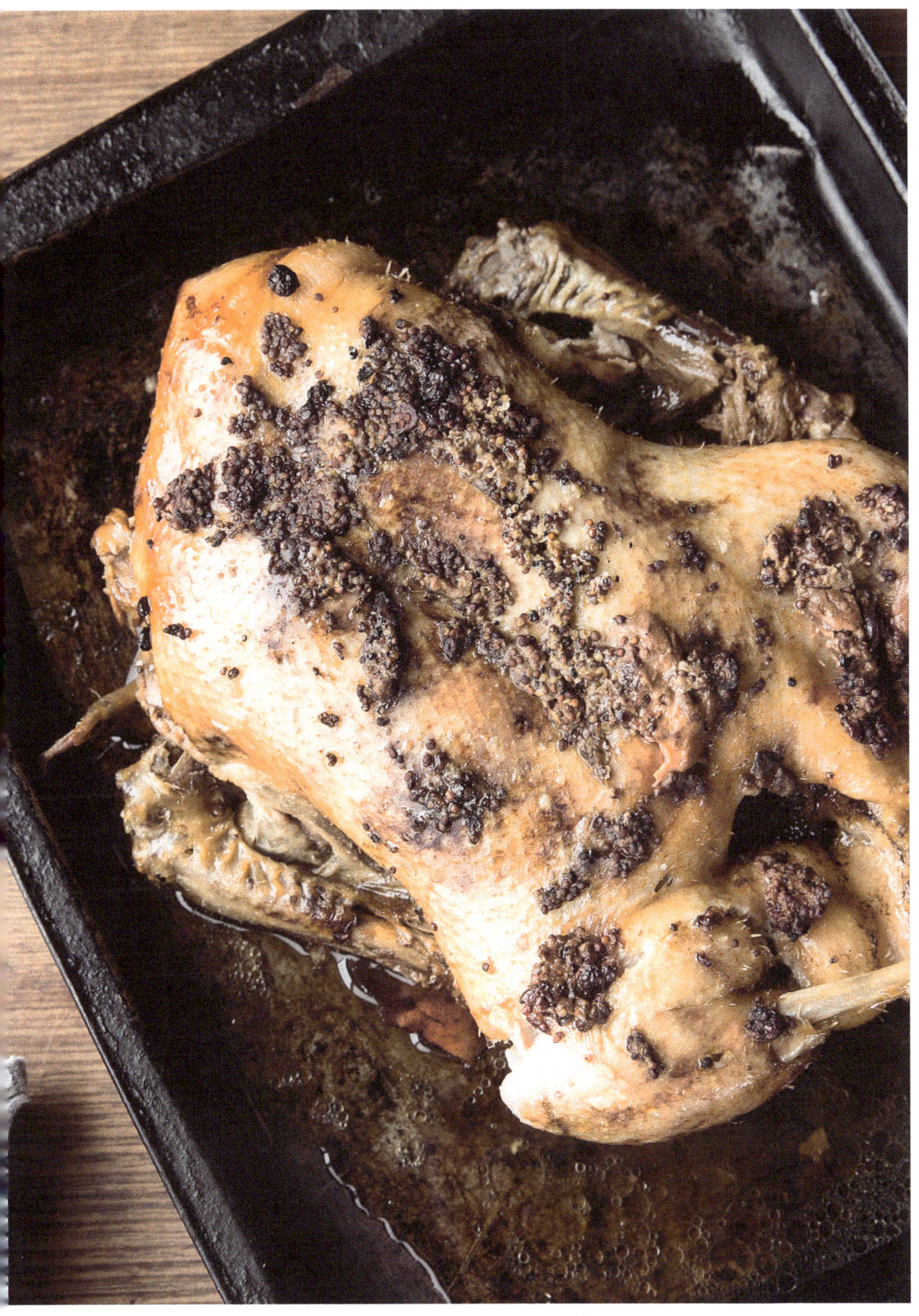

GRACE NIEUWENHUIZEN - MADE AT MARION

Italian Amaretti Biscuits

MAKES 12

Amaretti are traditional Italian biscuits. They are small, sweet and crunchy – a perfect accompaniment to a good coffee. These sweet bursts are gluten free and use up egg whites that you can't quite bring yourself to throw away. They take minutes to whip up and bake while I'm doing the dishes. When baking, you are aiming for a biscuit that is crisp on the outside, and soft in the middle. These biscuits are best eaten within the week.

1 cup almond meal

½ cup sugar

1 egg white

⅛ teaspoon almond extract

Almond slivers to decorate

Preheat the oven to 150°C.

Combine all ingredients in a large bowl and mix well until a stiff dough forms. Roll walnut size pieces into a ball and flatten into a round disc, approximately 1cm thick. Press an almond sliver into the centre of each disc and place on a tray lined with baking paper.

Bake in the oven for 23 minutes, or until just golden. Allow the amaretti to cool completely before removing from the tray.

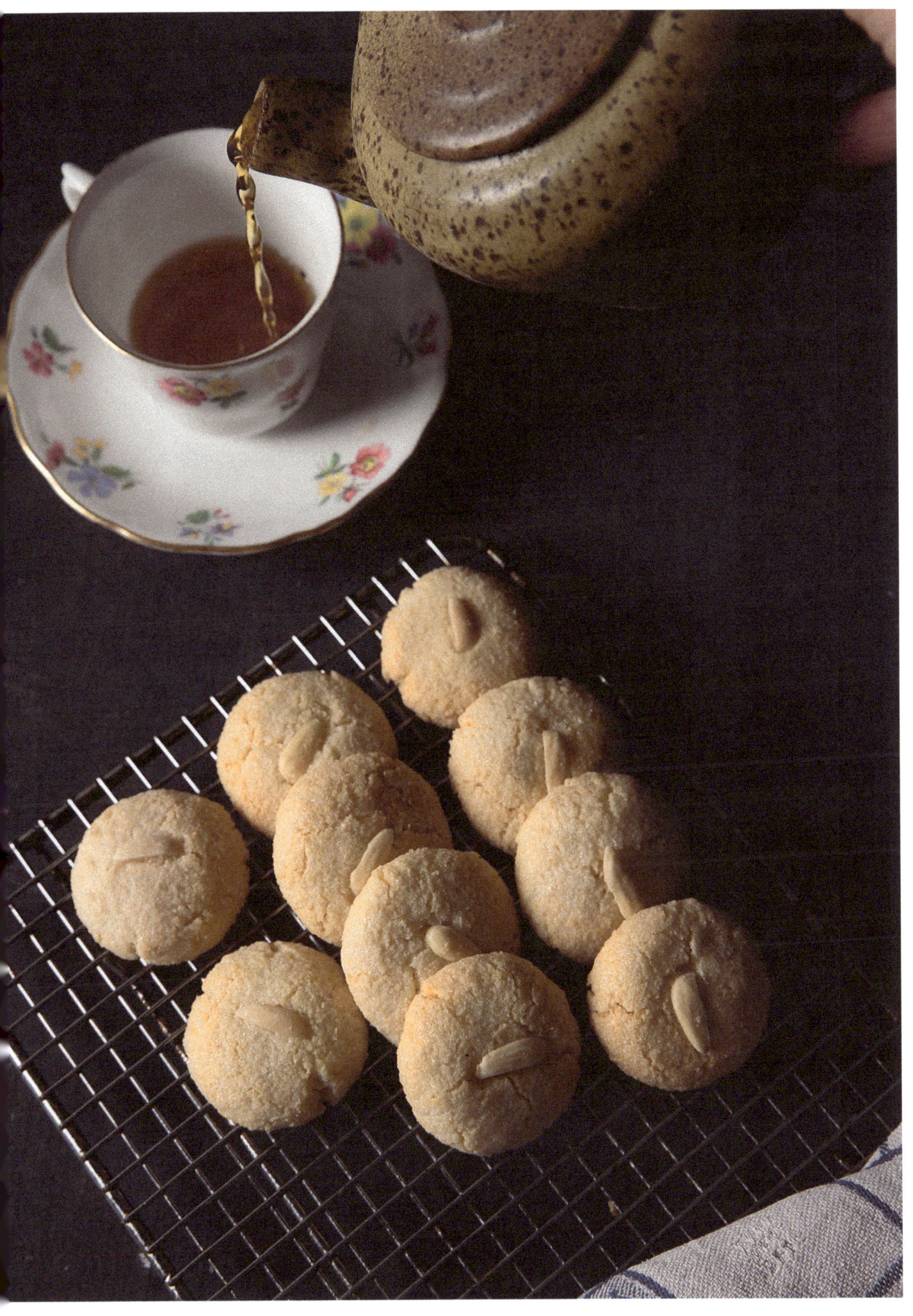

Butter Chicken and Naan Bread

SERVES 4-6

This is a very mild curry that is great for the whole family on cold winter nights. To make it even milder, leave the chilli out completely and use less tandoori paste. Serve it with basmati rice and nann bread.

MARINADE

600 grams chicken thigh fillets

200ml natural yoghurt

½ teaspoon cumin

1 teaspoon garam masala

1 tablespoon lemon juice

SAUCE

1 onion

2cm piece of ginger

1 green chilli

60g unsalted butter

3 cardamom pods

½ teaspoon paprika

½ teaspoon garam masala

¼ teaspoon cumin

¼ teaspoon coriander seed

400 grams chopped tomatoes

200ml chicken stock

100m cream

2 tablespoons coriander leaves

salt and pepper

NAAN BREAD

MAKES 6

450 grams bread flour

2 teaspoons dried yeast

1 teaspoon salt

1 teaspoon sugar

185ml warm water

90 grams natural yoghurt

2 tablespoons extra virgin olive oil

extra ghee, butter or extra virgin olive oil for pan frying

To make the marinade, slice the chicken into strips, and combine in a bowl with the combine the yoghurt, cumin, garam marsala, lemon juice and a pinch of salt. Stir well and refrigerate for at least 20 minutes or for a few hours.

To make the sauce, peel the onion and ginger, and remove the seeds from the chilli. Process in a food processor to make a paste.

Melt half of the butter in a deep frying pan over medium heat, add the cardamom pods, paprika, garam marsala, cumin, coriander and a pinch of salt and cook for 1 minute. Add the onion mixture and cook, stirring, for 5 minutes. Stir in the tomatoes and stock, cover and simmer gently for 15 minutes. Remove from the heat, allow to cool slightly, then transfer to a food processor and process until smooth. Return the sauce to the frying pan, add the chicken and simmer gently over medium heat for 15-20 minutes, or until the chicken is cooked. Add the cream, coriander leaves and the remaining butter and stir. Serve with rice and naan bread.

This is a recipe for plain naan bread, but if you want to add a bit of flavor you can press crushed garlic into one side of the bread before cooking, or once cooked you can top with grated cheese and pop into a hot oven for a minute or so until the cheese is melted.

Combine the flour, yeast, salt and sugar in a large bowl. Mix in the water, yoghurt and extra virgin olive oil. Knead the dough for 5 minutes or until smooth. Place dough in an oiled bowl, cover with plastic wrap and set aside in a warm place for 1 hour, or until the dough has doubled in size.

Punch down the dough and knead lightly. Divide the dough into six portions. Roll each into a tight ball then use a rolling pin to flatten into a disc about 20cm in diameter. Heat a frying pan over medium heat, add a splash of extra virgin olive oil and a knob of butter or ghee and cook each piece of naan for 2 minutes on each side, or until cooked through.

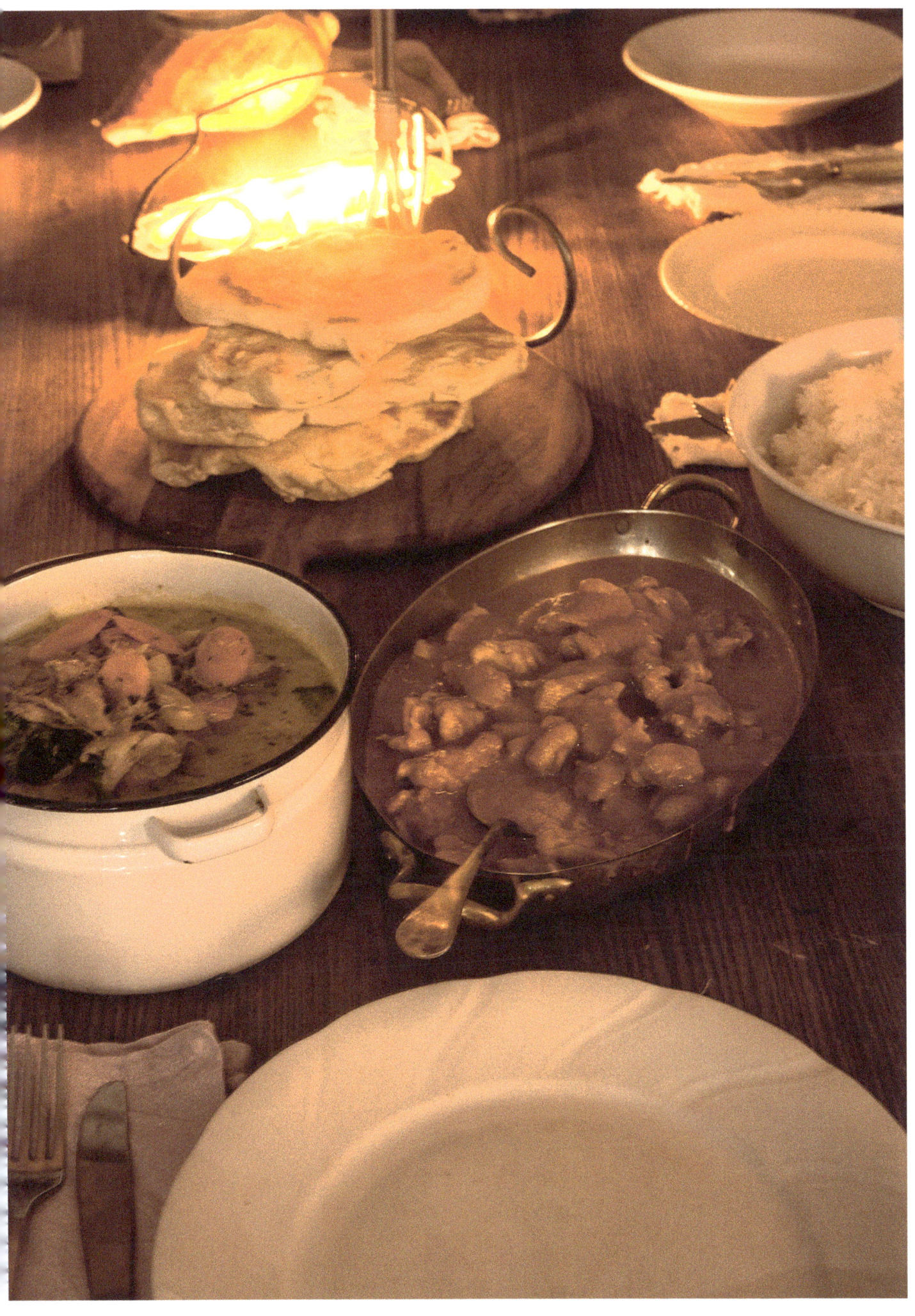

Crispy Baked Chicken Drumsticks

SERVES 6

It's lucky that children love drumsticks as they are a very economical choice for a family meal!

2 eggs

1 ½ cups plain flour

1 tablespoon smoked paprika

1 tablespoon oregano

1 teaspoon salt

1 teaspoon pepper

2-3 tablespoons extra virgin olive oil

1 kilogram chicken drumsticks

Preheat the oven to 170°C.

Crack the eggs into a large bowl and whisk with a fork until well combined. In a separate bowl, mix the flour with the paprika, oregano, and salt and pepper.

Pour the oil into a baking tray large enough to fit the drumsticks without them touching. Heat the baking tray in the oven for about 4 minutes, or until the oil is hot.

Coat each drumstick by dipping in egg, then rolling in flour. Repeat with all of the drumsticks. Lay the drumsticks in the baking try without them touching each other.

Bake in the oven for 35 - 40 minutes, turning once during the cooking time – try to avoid turning more than once so that the skin remains intact.

Serve with steamed veggies and mash, or with your favourite salad.

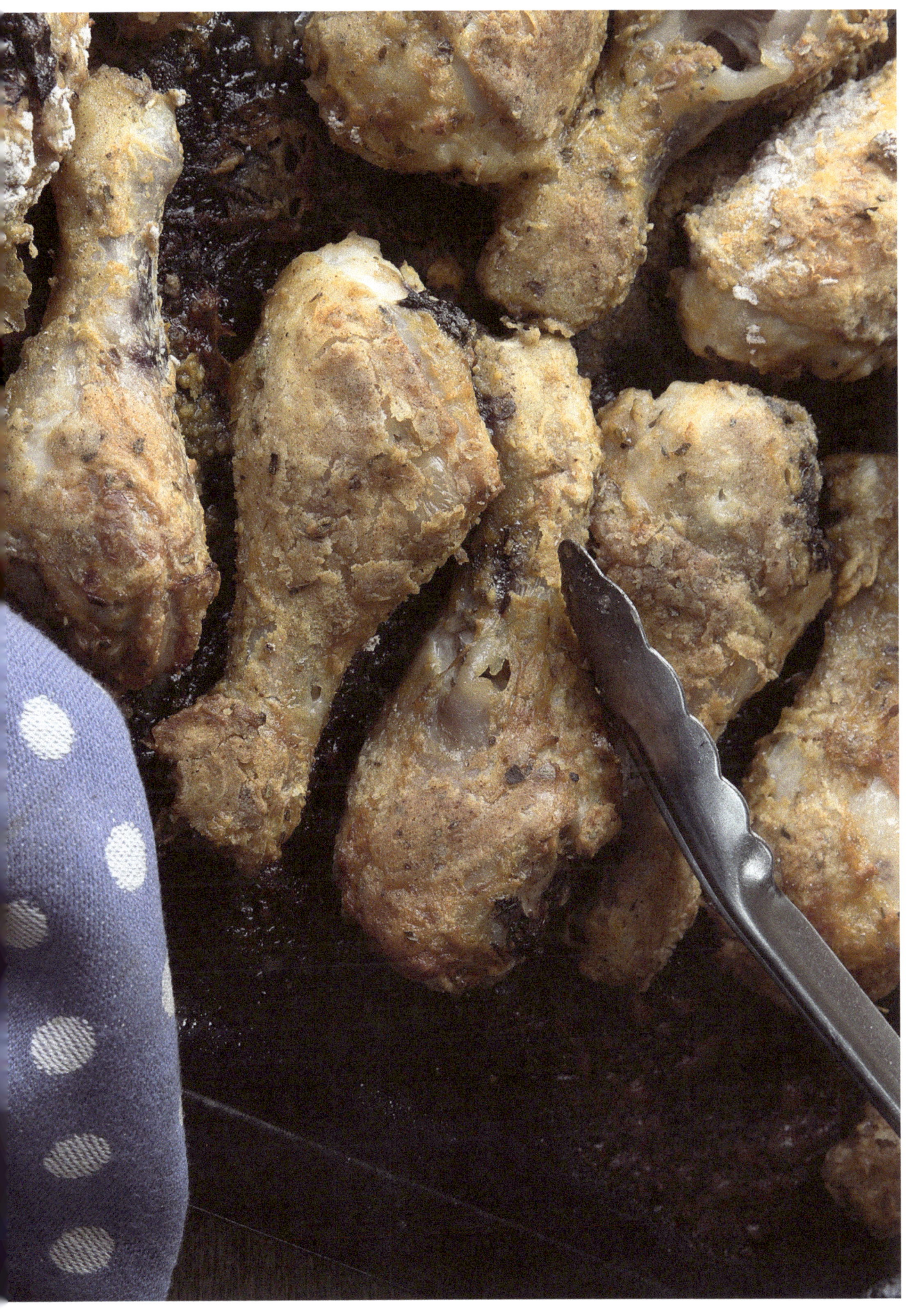

NIC DERKLEY - LUFRA HOTEL AND APARTMENTS

Fried Sichuan Quail with Strawberry Chilli Sauce

SERVES 4

This crispy, spicy quail is a great starter or entrée for a dinner party.

4 x Rannoch quail, boned and butterflied

MARINADE

1 teaspoon garlic

1 teaspoon ginger

4 tablespoons soy sauce

1 tablespoon rice wine vinegar

1 tablespoon Chinese cooking wine

STRAWBERRY CHILLI SAUCE

1cm knob ginger

2-4 long red chillies

2 garlic cloves

500 grams of fresh strawberries

⅓ cup of brown sugar

4 tablespoons of rice wine vinegar

QUAIL SEASONING

½ cup of corn flour

1 tablespoon of ground Sichuan pepper

1 tablespoon of sea salt

1 tablespoon Chinese 5 spice

½ teaspoon chilli powder

extra virgin olive oil - for frying

½ an iceberg lettuce

4 spring onions

To prepare the quail, cut each quail in half, and in half again so that you have two legs and two breasts per quail. Made a marinade by mixing together the garlic, ginger, soy sauce, rice vinegar and Chinese cooking wine and pour over quail. Marinate in the refrigerator for 2- 6 hours.

To make the sauce, finely chop the ginger and chillies, and crush the garlic. Heat a tablespoon of extra virgin olive oil over medium heat and sauté the garlic, ginger and chilli for 1-2 minutes. Add the strawberries and cook for 4 more minutes. Add the brown sugar and stir until it dissolves. Add the vinegar, reduce the heat to low and cook for 5 -10 minutes, or until the sauce reduces and thickens. Remove from the heat and pass the sauce through a fine sieve. Taste for seasoning – the sauce should be sweet and spicy with a zing of ginger.

Make the quail seasoning by mixing the cornflour, Sichuan pepper, sea salt, five spice and chilli powder.

To cook the quail, place a heavy-based frying pan over medium heat and fill with extra virgin olive oil to 1cm in depth and heat to 180C. Dust the quail pieces in the seasoning mix and carefully lower into the hot oil. You may need to cook the quail in small batches to avoid the temperature of the oil dropping. Cook, turning a couple of times, for approximately 45 seconds per side, or until crisp and golden. Remove from the oil and drain on paper towel.

To serve, shred the lettuce and finely chop the spring onions. Arrange the lettuce on the plates, place quail on top, sprinkle over the spring onions and drizzle with sauce. Offer extra sauce for dipping.

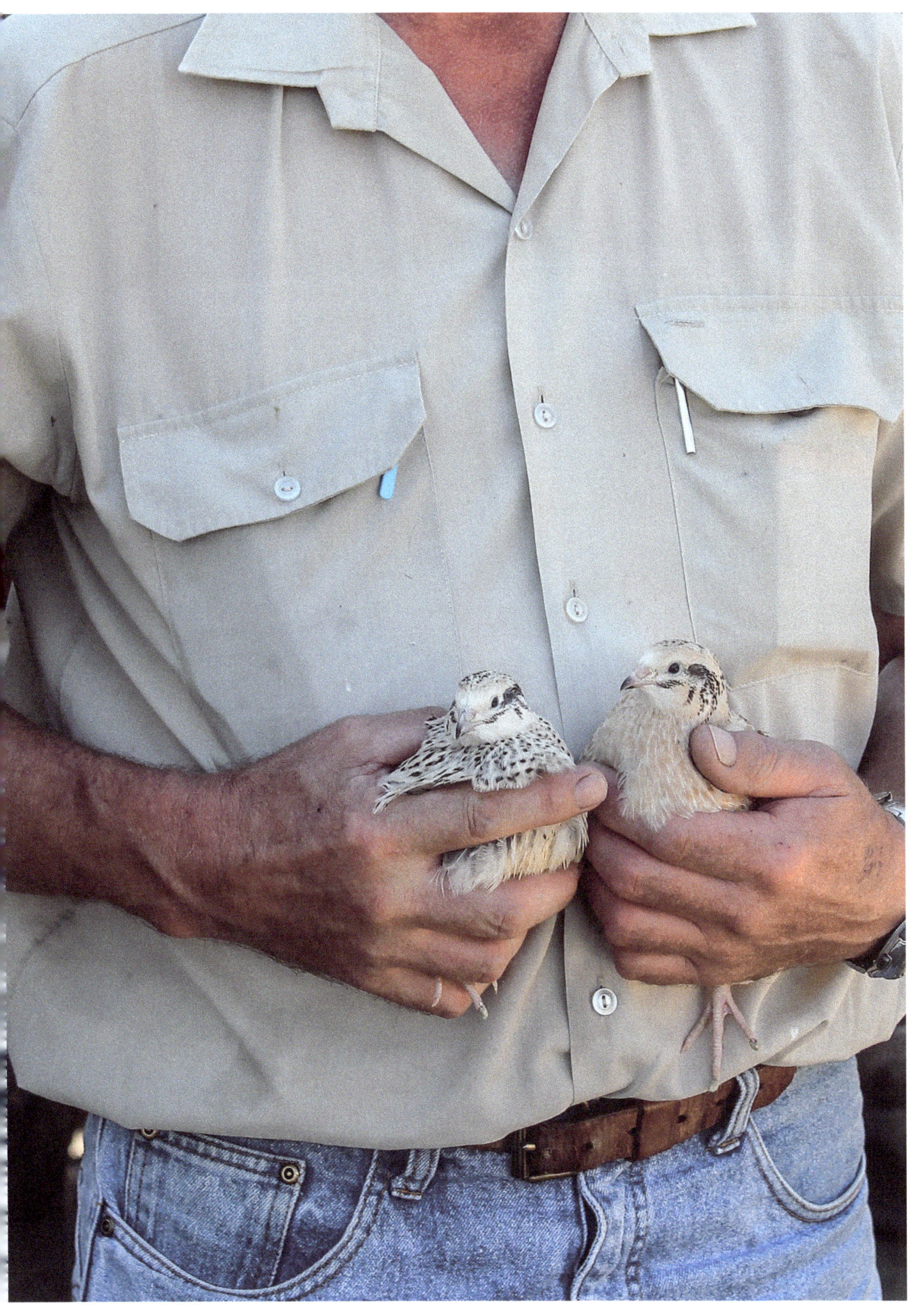

Hoi Sin Duck Breast with Beetroot Marmalade and Honey Roasted Parsnips

SERVES 4

This beautiful dish makes the most of fresh, locally sourced ingredients. To get the best flavour from the duck, marinate the duck breasts overnight in the fridge. If duck breast is not available, venison also works well with these flavours. To can buy pre-made duck jus at gourmet food stores, or find a recipe to make your own at www.eloiseemmett.com

4 duck breasts

MARINADE

4 cloves garlic

2 sticks lemongrass

4 teaspoons soy sauce

2 tablespoons hoisin sauce

200ml extra virgin olive oil

BEETROOT MARMALADE

8 beetroots

4 red onions

200ml extra virgin olive oil

2 teaspoons Chinese five spice

2 teaspoons turmeric

8 star anise

2 teaspoons chilli flakes

2 teaspoons honey

2 teaspoons redcurrant jelly

200 grams fresh raspberry jam

PARSNIPS

8 parsnips

200ml Tasmanian leatherwood honey

knob of butter

400 grams spinach or kale

200 grams butter

200ml duck jus

salt and pepper

To marinate the duck, score the fat of the duck breast using a sharp knife. Crush the garlic, finely slice the lemongrass and mix together with the soy and hoisin sauces, and extra virgin olive oil. Pour over the scored duck breast and refrigerate overnight.

To make the beetroot marmalade, peel and finely shred the beetroot, and thinly slice the red onion. Heat the extra virgin olive oil in a medium sized saucepan and sauté the beetroot and onion over medium heat for 40 minutes, or until softened. Add the Chinese five spice, turmeric, star anise and chilli flakes and fry for another minute, or until fragrant. Add the honey, redcurrant jelly and jam, bring to a simmer and cook slowly until it has reduced by half, or until the mixture starts to caramelise. Cover this sticky mixture with water and cook slowly until the liquid has almost reduced and you are left with a sticky marmalade.

To make the parsnips, preheat the oven to 180°C. Cut one parsnip into batons, dress with honey and season with salt and pepper. Tip into a baking tray and cook in the oven for 30 minutes or until golden – turning at least once during the cooking time. Make a parsnip puree with the other parsnip. Bring a saucepan of water to the boil, chop the parsnip, tip into the boiling water and cook for 25 minutes, or until soft. Blitz in the food processor with a knob of butter and season.

To cook the duck breast, heat a frying pan over medium-high heat. Cook the duck skin side down to render off some of the fat for 7 minutes, then turn and cook for a further 2 minutes. Remove from the heat and set aside to rest.

To cook the spinach, melt the butter in a small saucepan over medium heat, and cook until brown and nutty. Add the spinach and sauté quickly until wilted. Remove from the heat and drain on paper towel.

To serve, arrange the duck on the plate with the parsnip puree, roasted parsnips, spinach, beetroot marmalade and drizzle with warmed duck jus.

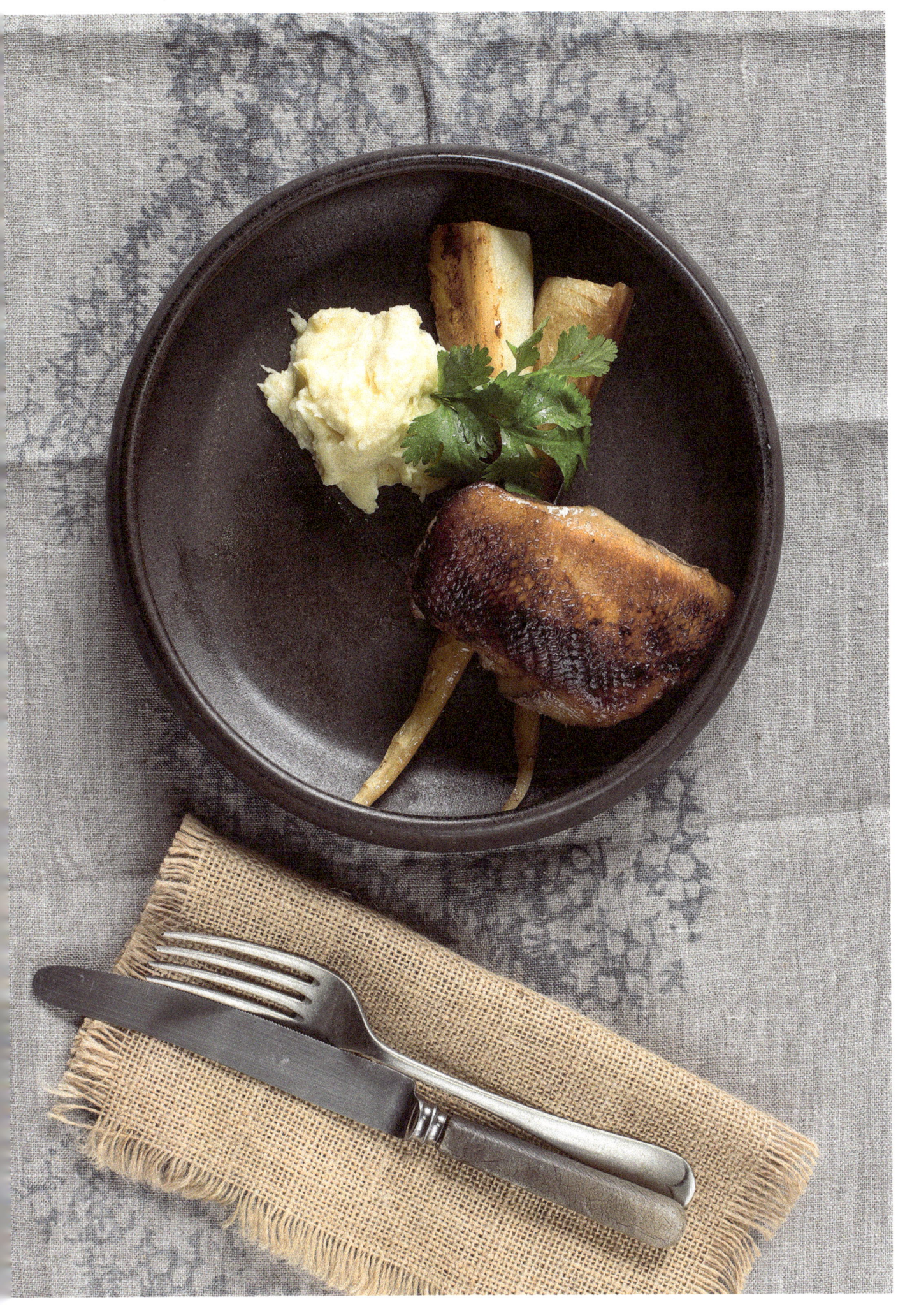

Quail with a Walnut, Blue Cheese and Apple Salad with a Honey Mustard Dressing

SERVES 4

DRESSING

20ml white wine vinegar

1 tablespoon honey

1 tablespoon Dijon mustard

40ml extra virgin olive oil

QUAIL

1 tablespoon extra virgin olive oil

4 quail (partially boned with leg and wing bone in and butterflied)

SALAD

150 grams of blue cheese

100 grams walnuts

2 medium apples

2 cups of salad leaves

To make the dressing, mix all ingredients together in a jar, and shake well to combine.

To cook the quail, preheat the oven to 180°C. Heat the oil in a oven-proof frying pan over high heat, season the quail and cook in the pan until sealed. Turn the butterflied quail skin side down put in the oven and cook for 10 minutes. Alternatively, you can use the barbecue to seal the quail, then cook on medium heat with the lid closed for 5-10 minutes.

To make the salad, roughly chop the walnuts and blue cheese and slice the apple. Toss together with the salad leaves and half of the dressing. Top the salad with the hot quail, drizzle over the remaining dressing and serve immediately.

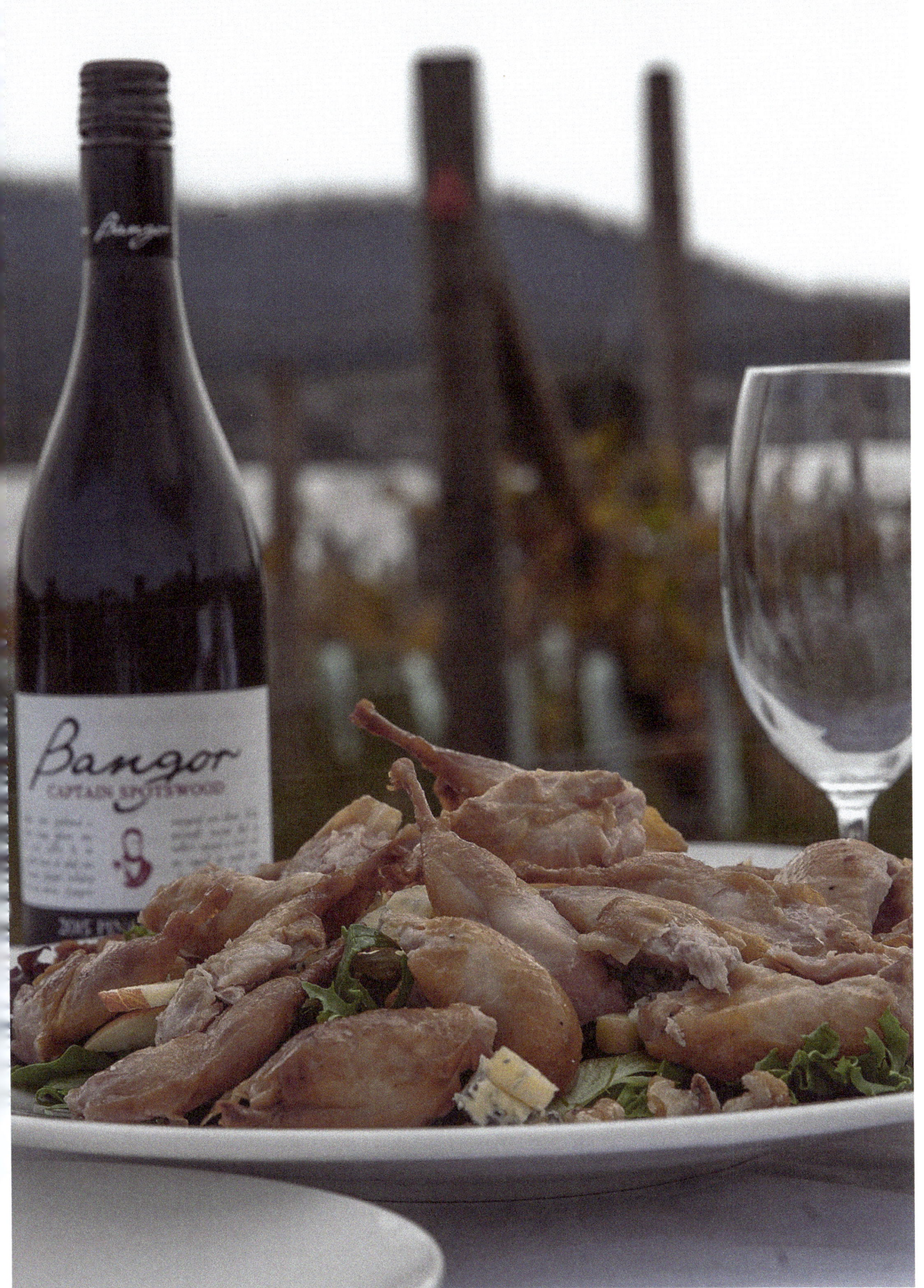

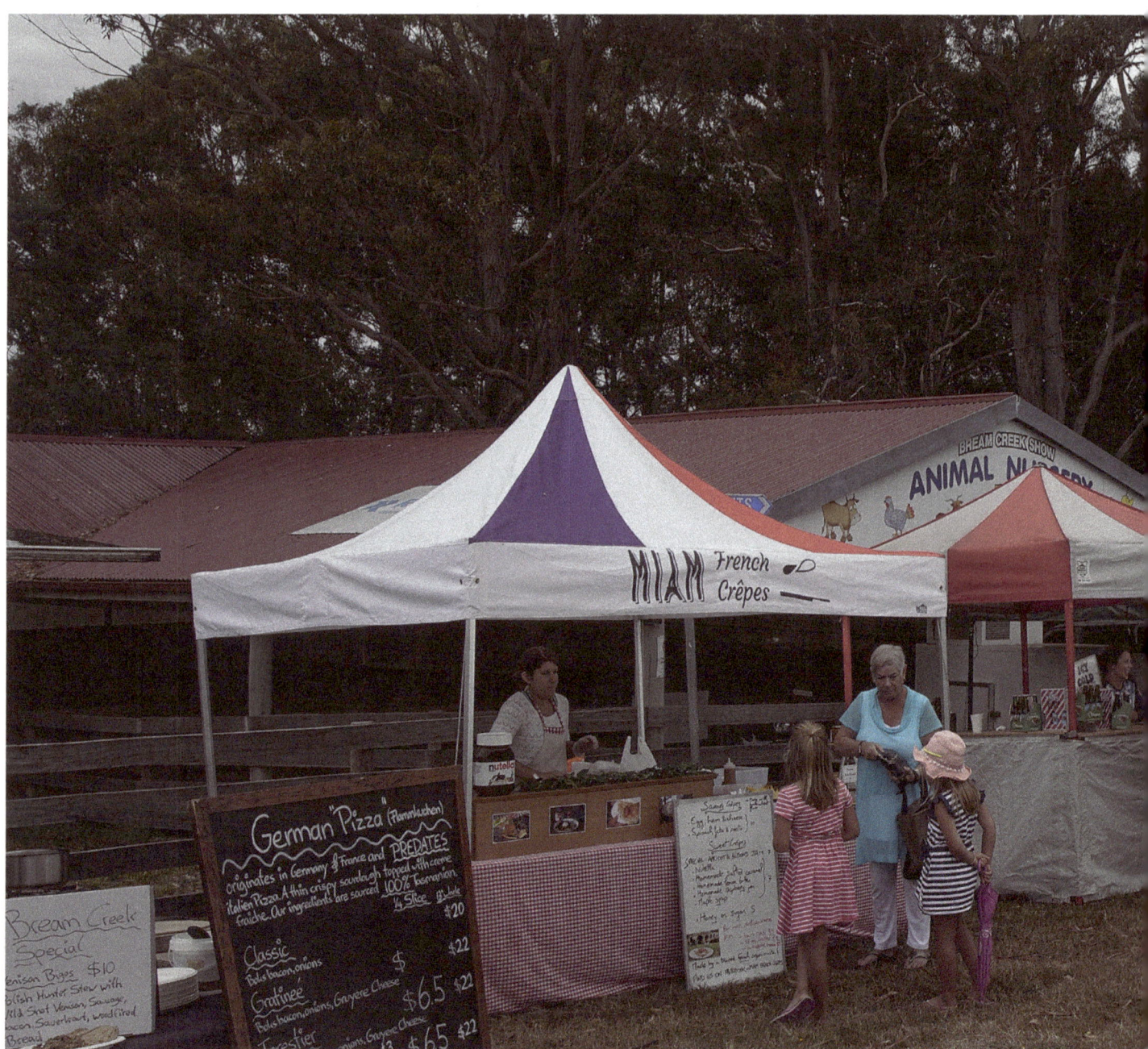

From the Dairy

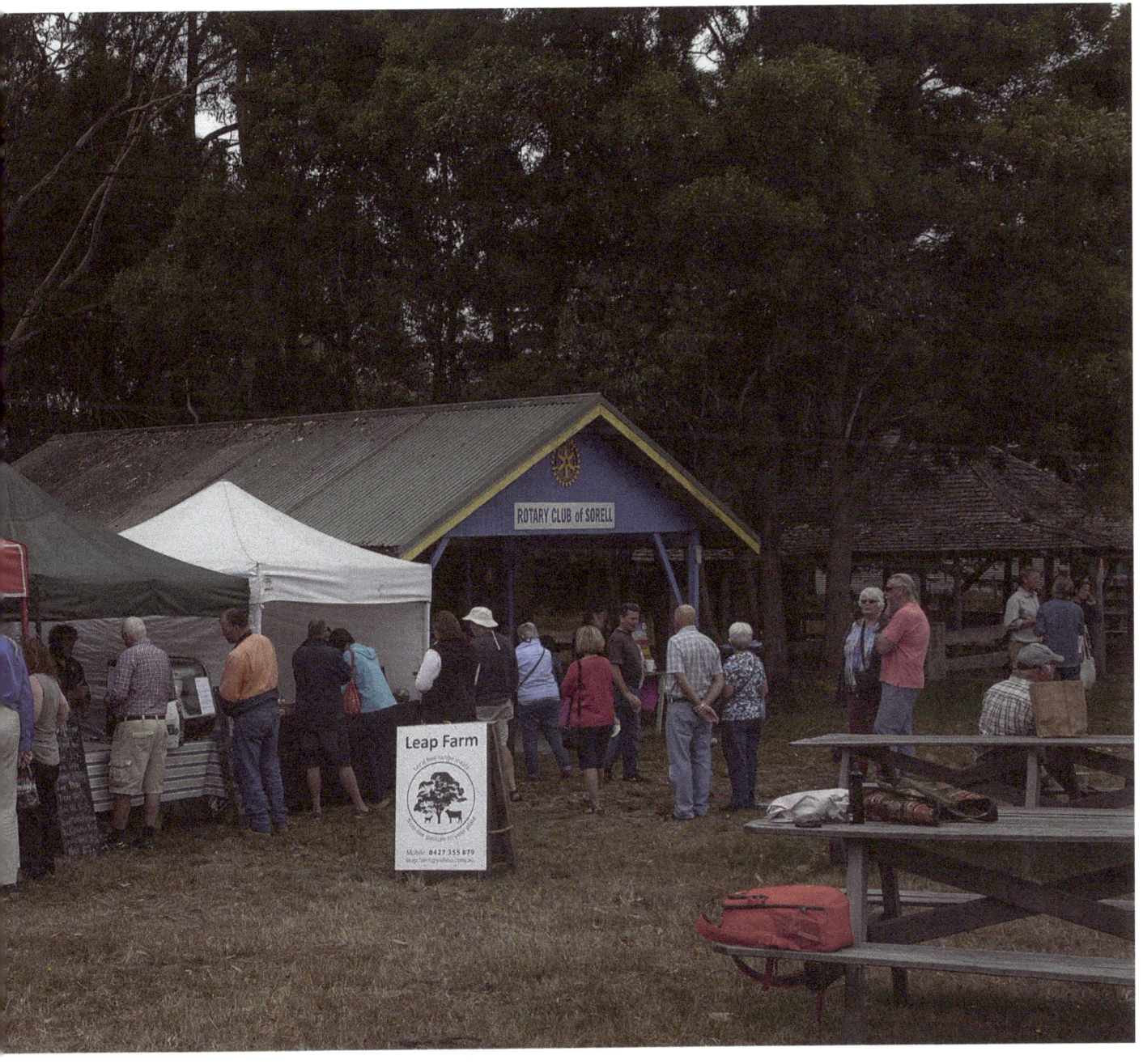

Rhubarb Clafoutis

SERVES 6

Clafoutis is a wonderful baked dessert with its origins in France. The fruit is surrounded by a thick batter, and the clafoutis is served warm with cream. Traditionally, pitted cherries are used, or you could try substituting fresh raspberries when in season. Although usually served as a dessert, clafoutis also makes a wonderful brunch dish.

1 tablespoon butter

2 tablespoons caster sugar

250 grams rhubarb

100 grams plain flour, or almond meal

½ teaspoon baking powder

3 eggs

150 grams caster sugar

150 grams cream

150 grams milk

1 teaspoon vanilla extract, or seeds from 1 vanilla bean

icing sugar, for dusting

Preheat the oven to 200°C.

Soften the butter and use it to grease the inside of a 25cm round or rectangular ceramic baking dish, then sprinkle with the caster sugar.

Slice the rhubarb stalks into 1cm pieces and arrange in the bottom of the dish. Using a large bowl, whisk together the plain flour (or almond meal), baking powder, eggs, sugar, cream, milk and vanilla until well combined.

Pour this mixture over the rhubarb, and once the fruit has floated to the top, sprinkle with a little more caster sugar to further sweeten the rhubarb.

Bake in the oven for 30-35 minutes, or until puffy and golden. To serve, dust with icing sugar and offer thick cream.

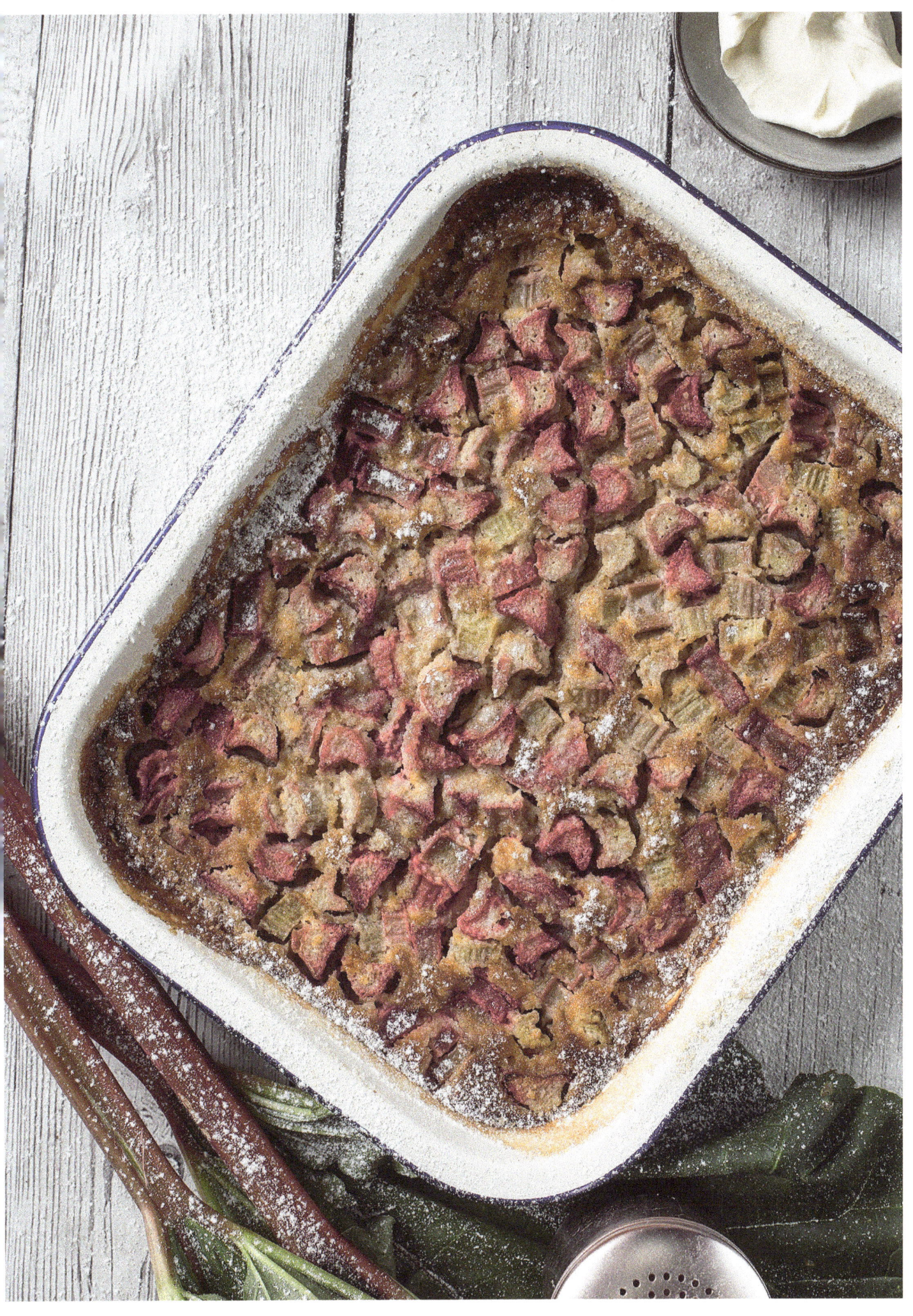

ARWEN GENGE - ARWEN'S THERMO PICS

Black Forest Trifle

SERVES 12

This trifle is a spectacular party dish. Most of the elements can be made the day before, but the cream is best whipped on the day it is served. To cut down on preparation time, you can make and freeze the chocolate sponge in advance, or use a bought chocolate cake instead. If you enjoy preserving fruit, it's well worth a trip to the cherry farm in summer to buy seconds, which you can then bottle yourself. Individual trifles can also be made – simply layer the ingredients into 8 individual glasses. Omit the kirsch for an alcohol-free dessert.

CHOCOLATE SPONGE

½ teaspoon bicarb soda

1 teaspoon cream of tartar

60 grams corn flour

30 grams cocoa powder

150 grams caster sugar

4 eggs, at room temperature

1 teaspoon vanilla extract

2 tablespoons hot water

CHERRY JELLY

1 x 600 gram jar preserved cherries (or use a jar of marello cherries)

2 teaspoons gelatine power

CHOCOLATE CUSTARD

1000 grams milk

100 grams cornflour

150 grams sugar, or to taste

4 eggs

2 teaspoons vanilla extract

150 grams dark chocolate

40 grams unsalted butter

TO ASSEMBLE

2 tablespoons kirsch - optional

1000 grams cream

100 grams flaked almonds or coconut flakes

50 grams dark chocolate

To make the chocolate sponge, preheat the oven to 180°C. Grease and line a 25cm cake tin. Using a large bowl, sift together the bicarbonate of soda, cream of tartar, cocoa and cornflour and set aside. Separate the eggs and beat the whites in a clean bowl using an electric mixer, for 2- 4 minutes, or until stiff peaks form. With the beaters still running, add the sugar one teaspoon at a time, and beat until well incorporated – don't rush this process, it will take 4-5 minutes. Gently fold the yolks into the whipped egg whites, one yolk at a time. Using a spatula, fold the vanilla, hot water and cornflour mixture through the beaten egg mixture. Pour into the prepared tin and bake for 35-40 minutes or until an inserted skewer comes out clean. Turn out onto a wire rack to cool completely before using.

To make the cherry jelly, drain the cherries, reserving the liquid. If you are using Kirsch, pour it over the drained cherries to infuse, and set aside. Using a small saucepan, heat 100ml of the cherry liquid over low heat, add the gelatine and stir until dissolved. Add the remainder of the cherry liquid and stir to combine. Strain this liquid through a sieve and pour into the base of the trifle bowl, or pour equal amounts into the 8 individual dishes. Carefully drop the cherries into the jelly mixture and put into the refrigerator to set. (Some people like to add the chocolate sponge at this point, which allows it to soak up the jelly mixture, then top with the cherries – the choice is up to you!)

To make the custard, pour the milk into a saucepan and bring to a simmer over low heat. Whisk the cornflour, sugar, eggs and vanilla in a large bowl, and pour in the hot milk. Whisk well, return to the saucepan, stirring continuously until the mixture thickens. Alternatively, use a Thermomix to make the custard. Add all of the custard ingredients to the bowl and cook for 15 minutes at 90°C on speed 4, or until the custard is thick. Set aside to cool.

Pour the cream into a bowl and whip using an electric mixer until soft peaks form. Refrigerate until required.

To assemble the trifle, break the chocolate cake and cover the cherry jelly with the pieces of cake (unless you've done so in an earlier step). Top with a layer of drained cherries. Pour in the custard layer and put into the refrigerator to cool. Once fully chilled, spread the top with whipped cream.

To decorate, sprinkle with lightly toasted, flaked almonds and grated dark chocolate, or with toasted coconut flakes and fresh cherries or seasonal berries.

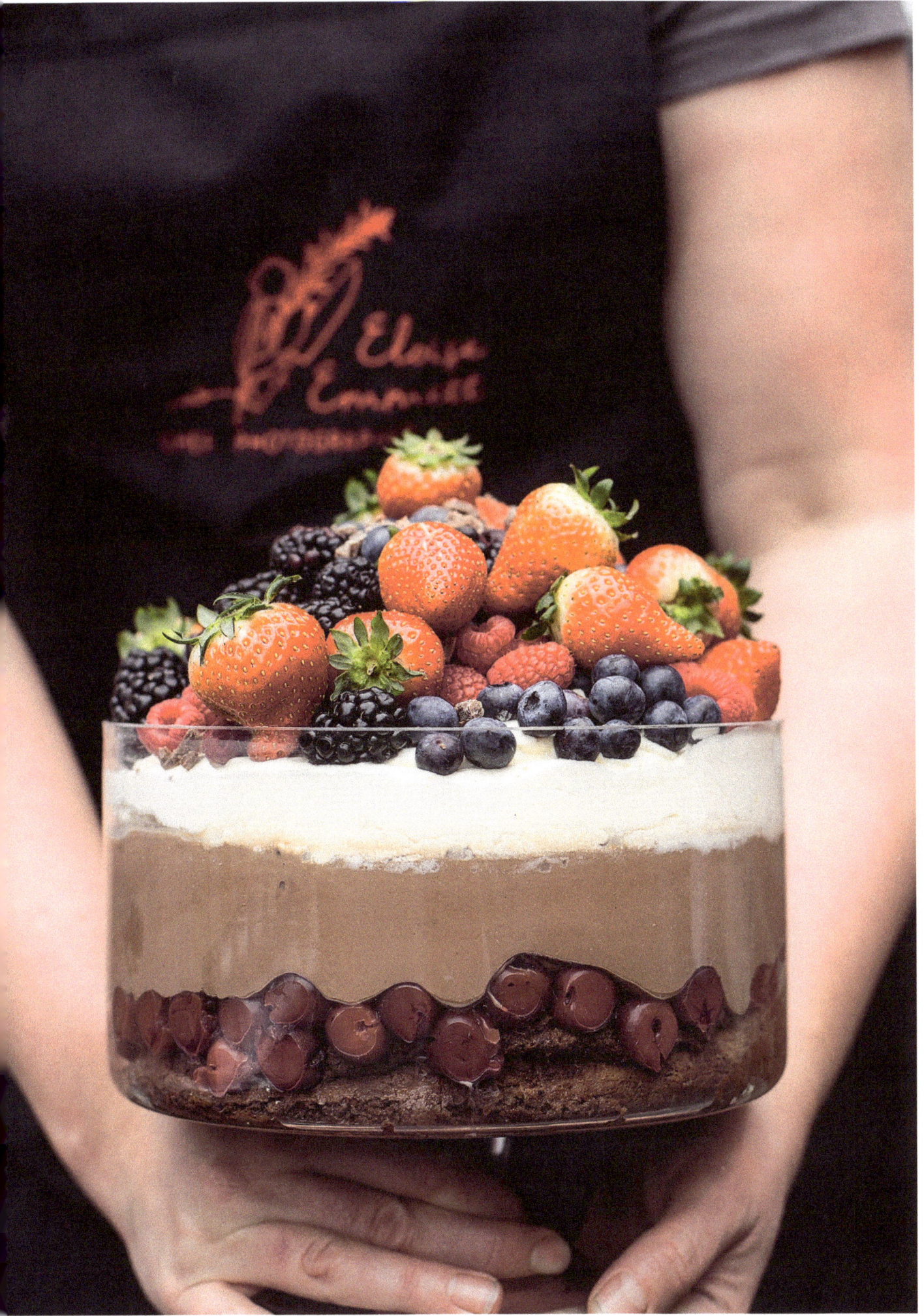

KATE FIELD - TONGOLA DAIRY

Mushroom Pasta with Billy Goat Cheese

SERVES 4

Tongola Billy is a washed rind goat cheese with a nutty flavour that pairs very well with the mushrooms and thyme in this easy pasta dish. Instead of grating the cheese, you may prefer to dice it into small chunks so that it doesn't melt completely. If you prefer, you can create a creamy sauce by adding in 100g of Curdy (or fresh goat's Chevre) instead of the Billy. To make your own fresh pasta, see page 158 or use a packet of dried pasta instead.

40 grams butter

4 large Swiss brown mushrooms

4 large button mushrooms

4 cloves garlic

1 tablespoon dried thyme

300 grams fresh pasta

50 grams of Tongola Billy goat cheese

salt and pepper

To make the sauce, melt the butter in a large frying pan over low heat. Roughly chop the mushrooms and fry in the butter for 3-5 minutes or until softened and brown. Finely chop the garlic and add to the pan, and stir in the thyme.

Bring a large saucepan of salted water to the boil, drop in the fresh pasta and cook until al dente. Drain off the water and return the pasta to the saucepan. Add the mushroom mixture and stir to combine.

Grate the Billy goat cheese and stir through the pasta – you may need to return the saucepan to a low heat and stir gently to help melt the cheese.

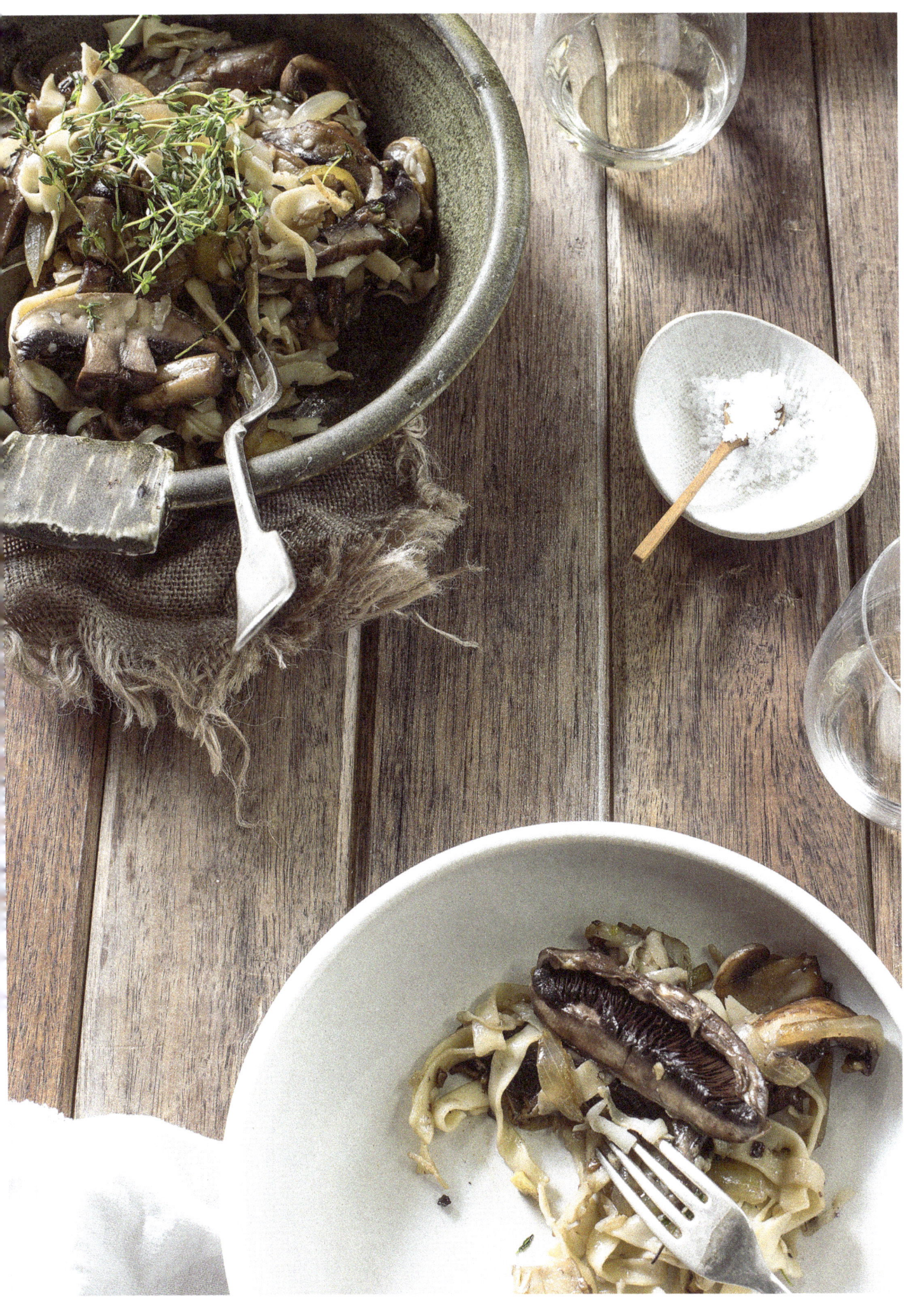

KATE FIELD - TONGOLA DAIRY

Tongola Pea Pasta

SERVES 4

This recipe is a great option when you want delicious food, but it needs to be quick, easy and with limited cleaning up required! The recipe for fresh homemade pasta is on page 158, alternatively use a packet of pasta and add the peas and beans to the pasta for the final five minutes of cooking time. Substitute fresh goat cherve for the Curdy if required.

300 grams fresh pasta

200 grams frozen peas

100 grams podded broad beans, fresh or frozen

1 clove of fresh garlic

50 grams grated cheddar cheese

150 grams Tongola Curdy goat cheese

salt and pepper

Bring a large saucepan of salted water to the boil, add the fresh pasta and return to the boil. Drop the peas and broad beans into the water to finish cooking with the pasta.

When the pasta is al dente, drain off the water and return the pea and pasta mixture to the saucepan. Finely chop the garlic, grate the cheddar and stir through the pasta, along with the Curdy cheese.

Season with salt and pepper to taste and serve immediately.

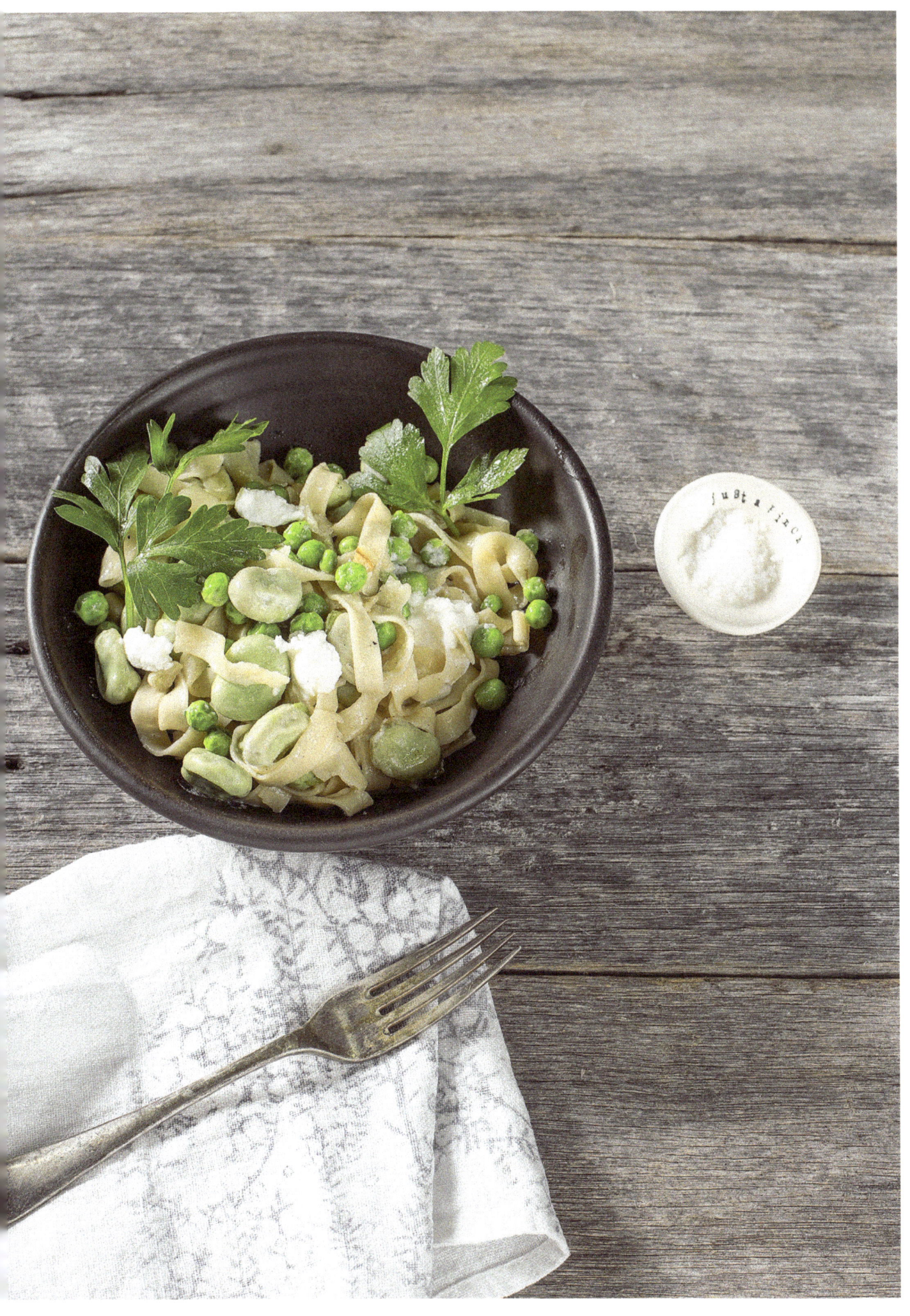

CLARE DEAN - PORT ARTHUR LAVENDER FARM

Fried Camembert Cheese with Strawberry and Lavender Coulis

SERVES 8 AS A CANAPÉ

CHEESE

200 gram wheel of Camembert cheese

2 tablespoons lavender flowers

1 cup plain flour

2 eggs

50ml milk

1 cup panko breadcrumbs

extra virgin olive oil for deep-frying

COULIS

250 grams strawberries

50 grams white sugar

75ml water

2ml lavender essential oil

1 tablespoon cornflour

To prepare the cheese, cut the wheel of Camembert into 8 equal portions. Grind the dried lavender flowers in a mortar and pestle and mix in a small bowl with the plain flour. Whisk the eggs and milk together in a small bowl and set aside.

Tip breadcrumbs onto a plate or small bowl. Roll each piece of cheese in the flour, dip into the egg mixture and roll in breadcrumbs. Set aside and repeat with the remaining pieces of cheese.

To make the coulis, remove the tops from the strawberries. Using a blender or food processor, blend the strawberries, sugar, cornflour and water until smooth.

Tip the mixture into a small saucepan and slowly bring to the boil over low heat, simmer for 15 minutes, until the sauce thickens. Set aside to cool and then stir through the lavender oil.

To cook the cheese, use a deep fryer set at 185°C. Cook the pieces of cheese for 60-90 seconds or until the coating is golden and the inside of the cheese is melted. To cook in the frying pan, heat one tablespoon of oil over medium-high heat and cook the pieces of cheese for 1-2 minutes on each side, or until golden all over.

Serve the hot cheese with the strawberry coulis as a dipping sauce.

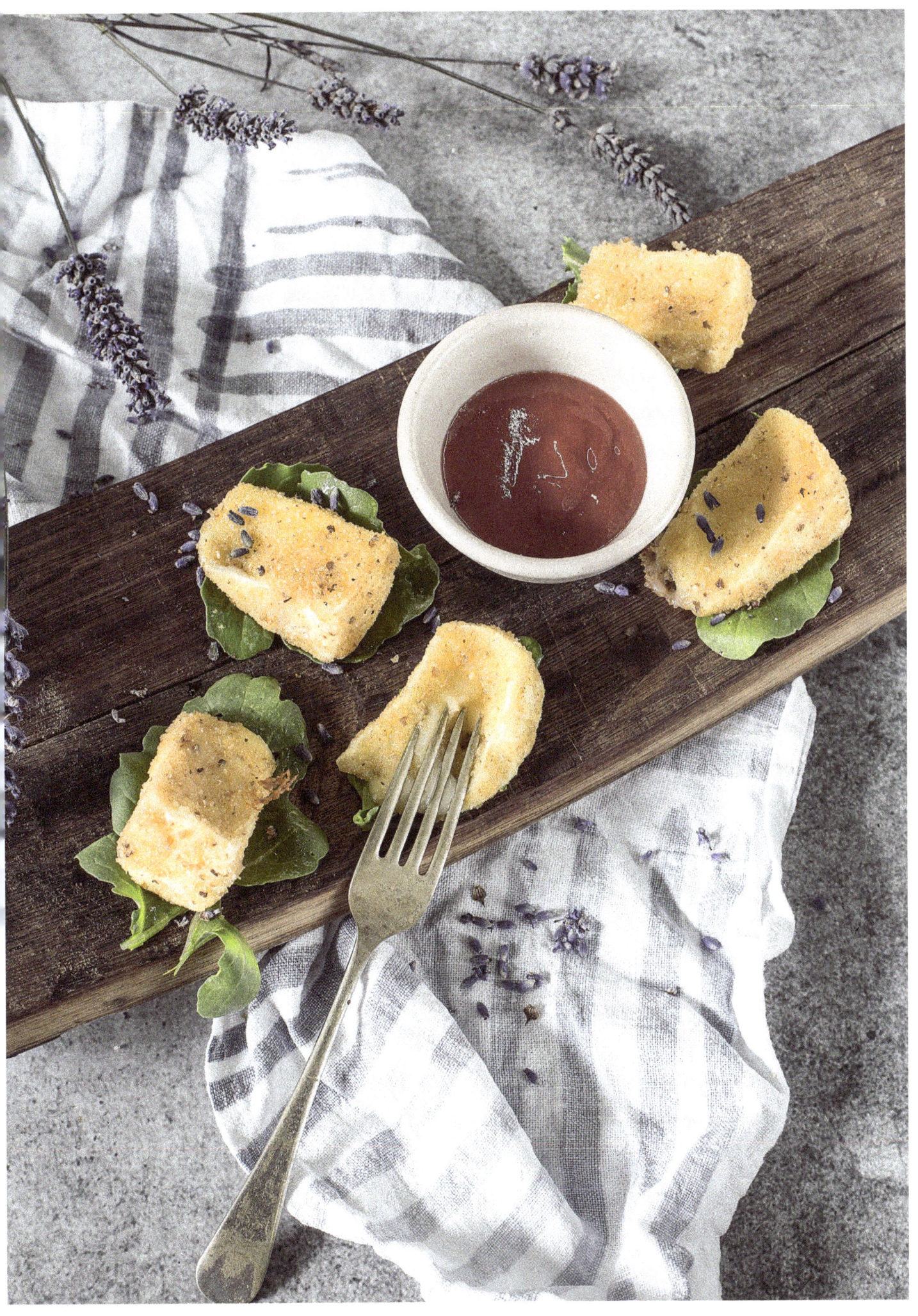

Blue Cheese, Pea and Prosciutto Risotto

SERVES 4

This flavoursome risotto is a meal in itself, but I also like to serve it alongside a grilled steak or chicken breast, or even a piece of fish. This is particularly delicious served with steak, and with a beef jus drizzled over the top.

1100ml chicken or vegetable stock

1 tablespoon butter

1 onion

2 cloves garlic

350 grams Arborio rice

100ml white wine

100 grams peas

100 grams prosciutto

30 grams Parmesan cheese

70 grams Gorgonzola cheese

a few sprigs of parsley and basil

Bring the stock to a gentle boil in a saucepan.

Using another large, heavy-based saucepan, melt the butter over medium heat. Finely dice the onion and crush the garlic, add to the pan and sauté for 3 minutes, or until tender. Add the rice and cook for one minute, stirring well.

Add the wine and stir. Gradually add the hot stock, one ladleful at a time, stirring regularly – wait until each ladle of stock is almost fully absorbed by the rice before adding the next. This process will take 15-20 minutes.

Cut/shred the prosciutto and dice the Gorgonzola cheese. Stir the cheese and prosciutto through the risotto and add the parsley and basil leaves.

Cover and set aside to rest for a few minutes to finish cooking, and then serve immediately.

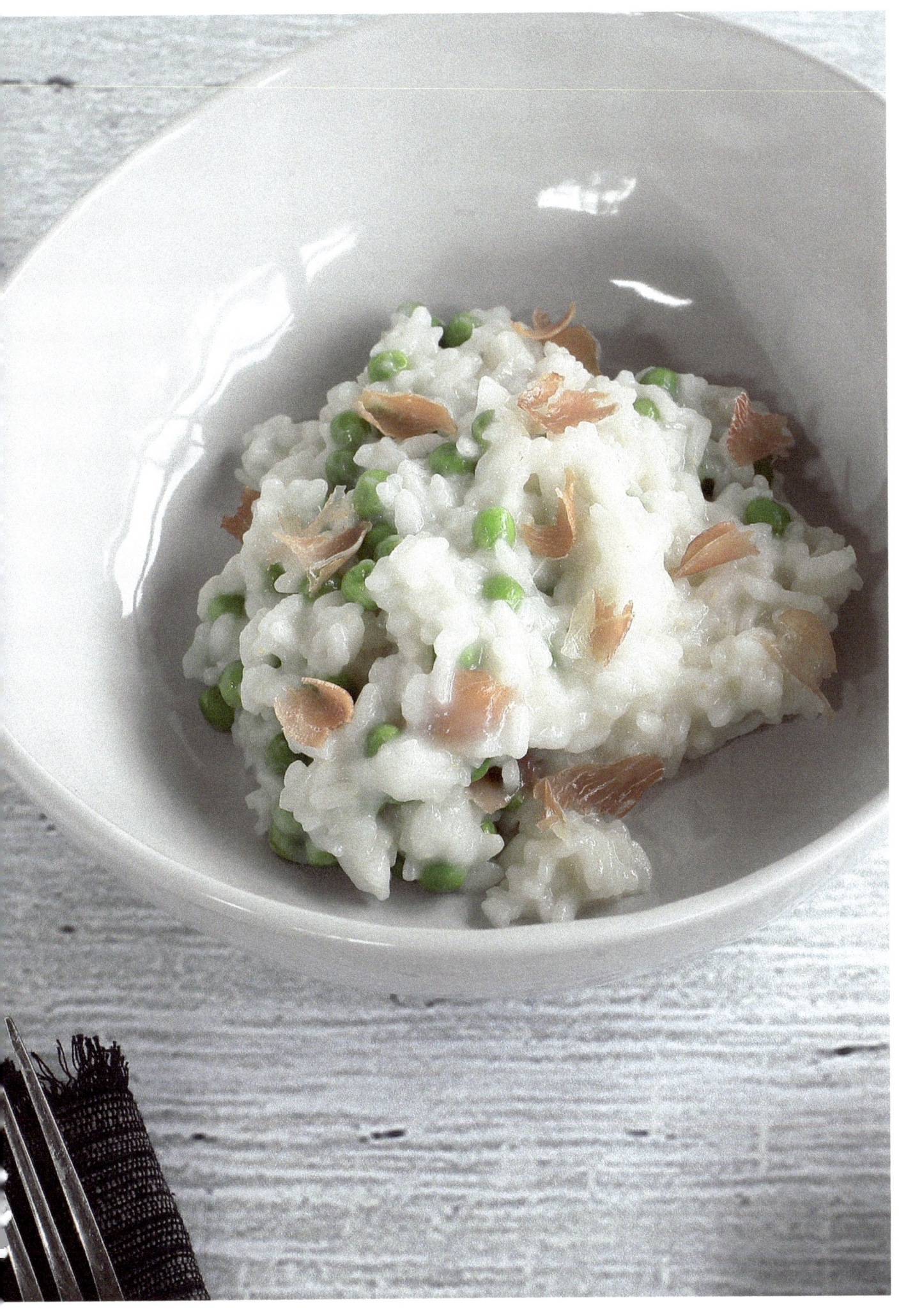

Kahlua and Baileys Chocolate Tart

SERVES 8

The combination of coffee, chocolate and whisky flavours in this tart are irresistible – it is such a delicious end to a special dinner. Serve with espresso coffee, or even espresso martinis for a big celebration!

BASE

240 grams plain flour

1 tablespoon sugar

180 grams butter

3 tablespoons water

FILLING

1 ½ cups white chocolate pieces

1 ½ cups milk chocolate pieces

1 ½ cups cream

60ml Baileys Irish Cream

60ml Kahlua liqueur

Preheat the oven to 180°C. Grease and flour a 20cm tart, flan or cake tin and set aside.

Use a food processor to make the base. Tip the flour and sugar into the processor, and with the motor still running, add the cubed butter. Process until the mixture resembles fine crumbs, add the water and process until the mixture comes together into a firm dough.

Alternatively, rub the butter into the flour and sugar with your fingers, then add the water and knead on a floured bench until the mixture comes together. Roll out the pastry to approximately 4mm thick, and line the base and sides of the prepared tin.

Set aside to rest for at least 30 minutes. Blind bake the base in the oven for 20 minutes, or until cooked through and golden. Leave to cool while you make the filling.

To make the two fillings, bring two saucepans of water to a simmer and place a bowl over each. Place the white chocolate into one bowl, and the milk chocolate into the other, add half the cream to each bowl and stir gently until melted and well combined.

Pour the Baileys into the white chocolate and the Kahlua into the milk chocolate into the other, and mix well. Pour the chocolate mixes into the base and swirl together lightly. Refrigerate for 2 hours, or until set, and serve.

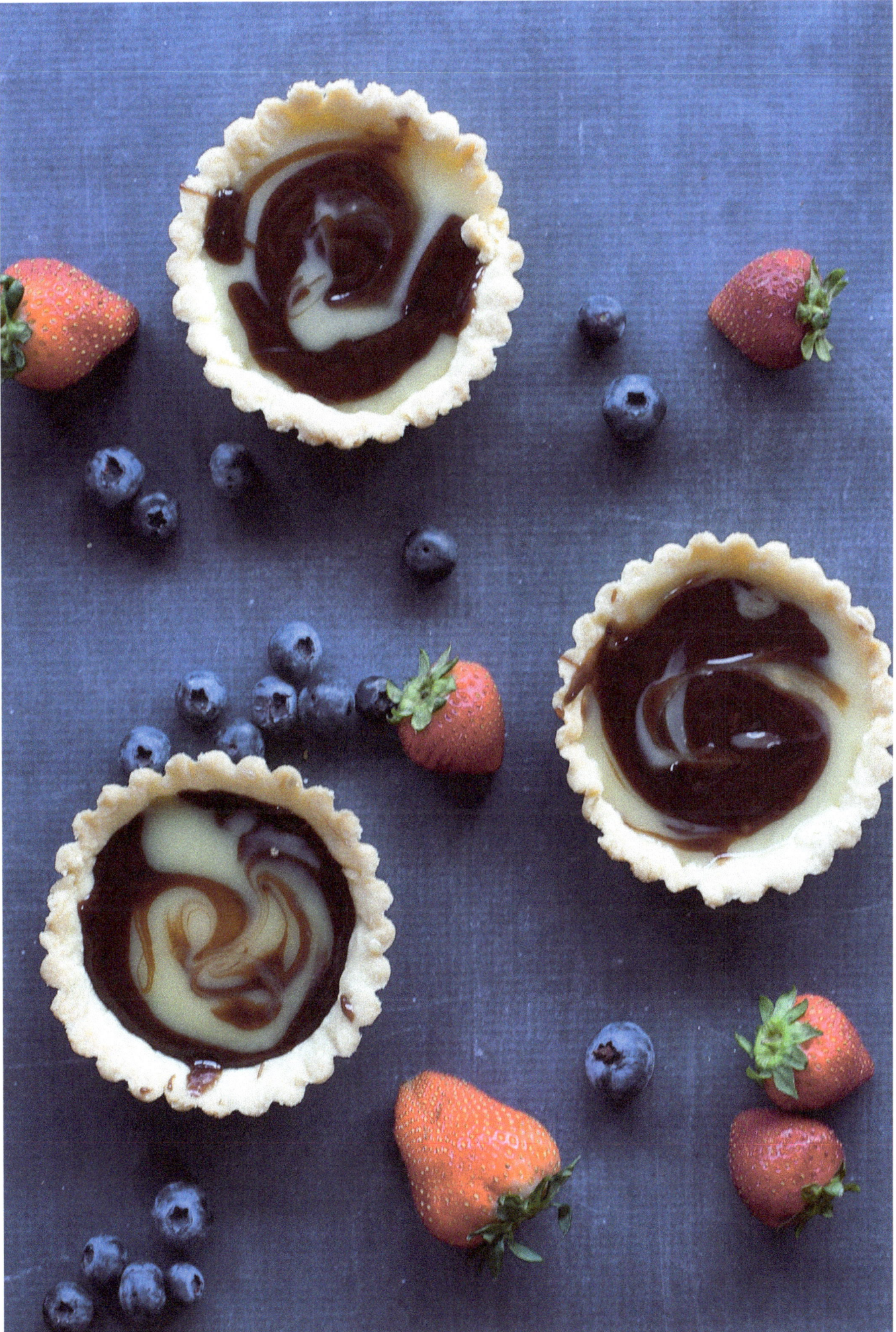

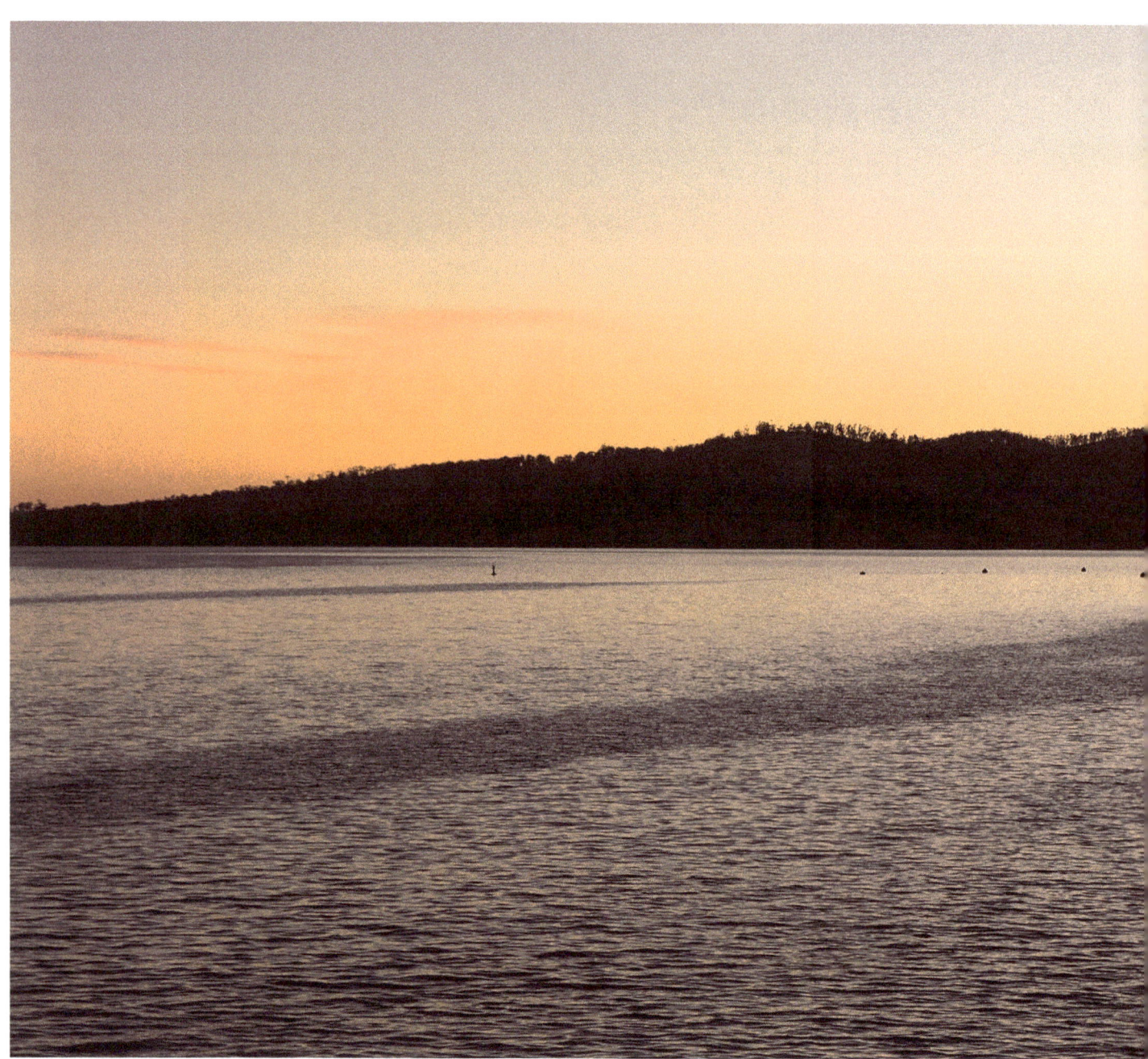

From the Sea Farm

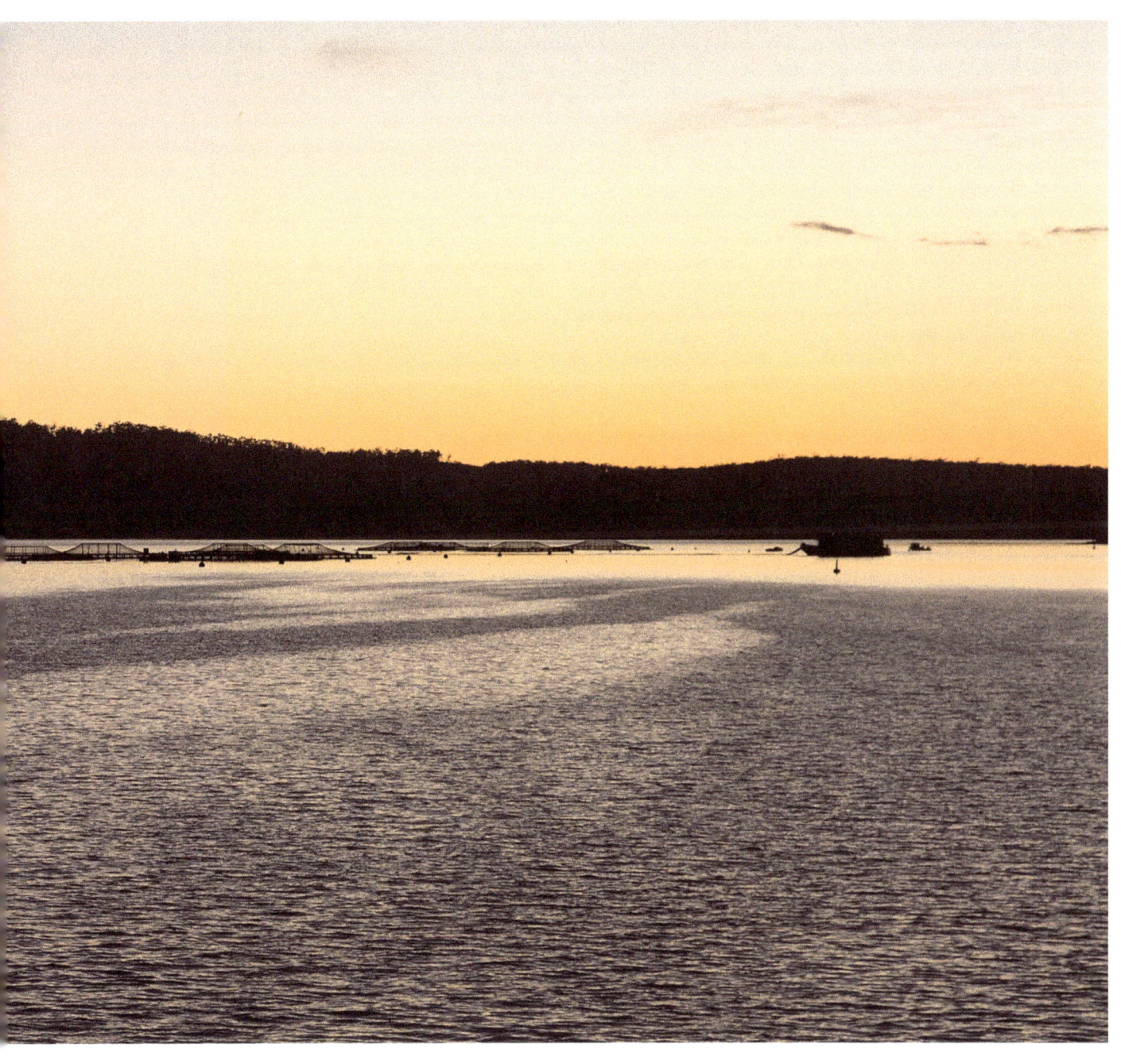

SUSAN CATCHPOLE - ROCKWALL BAR AND GRILL

Oysters with a Tangy Shallot Dressing

MAKES ENOUGH FOR 1-2 DOZEN OYSTERS

In Tasmania we are lucky to get oysters harvested on the same day as we serve them in the restaurant, and with oysters that fresh, they hardly need anything else! Natural oysters are always popular, so if you are serving them for a party, prepare a platter with rock salt (to stop the oysters moving around), arrange the oysters on top with some lemon or lime wedges and offer a bowl of this tangy dressing. Your guests can then choose how to have their oysters – natural, with a squeeze of lemon or lime, or drowned in this Asian-inspired sauce!

1 shallot

1 small red chilli

1 clove garlic

2 tablespoons rice wine vinegar

1 ½ tablespoons fish sauce

1 tablespoon palm sugar

1 teaspoon lemon juice

1-2 dozen oysters

Finely dice the shallot, finely chop the chilli and crush the garlic. Mix with the rice wine vinegar, fish sauce, palm sugar and lemon juice. Refrigerate until required to let the flavours develop.

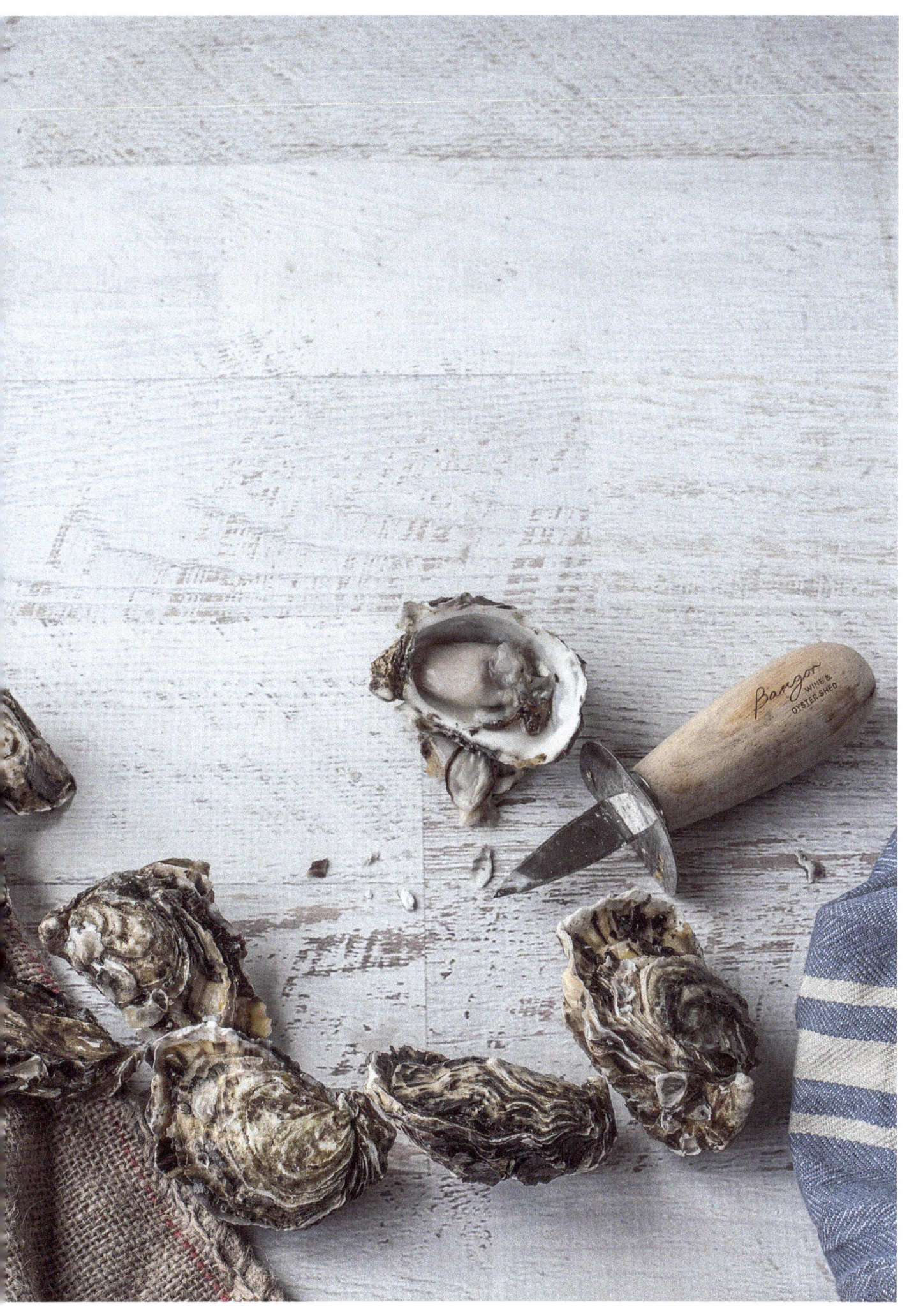

Petuna Ocean Trout with a Yoghurt Garlic Dressing and Pine Nut Herb Topping

SERVES 4-6

Ocean trout from Petuna is world renowned for it's intense colour, pure flavor and distinctive marbling. This delicate topping beautifully complements the creamy flavor of the fish.

1 kilo piece of Petuna Ocean Trout pin boned & skinned

extra virgin olive oil

salt and pepper

1 bunch rocket leaves

2 lemons

DRESSING

2 garlic cloves

75 grams natural yoghurt

2 teaspoons tahini

TOPPING

50 grams roasted pine nuts

½ cup parsley and mint

6 basil leaves

2 long red chilli

1 lemon

1 small Spanish onion

60ml extra virgin olive oil

Preheat the oven to 180°C.

Brush the ocean trout with extra virgin olive oil, sprinkle with salt, place on a baking tray and bake for 15 minutes.

Coat the unpeeled garlic cloves with a splash of extra virgin olive oil and roast in the oven for 10 minutes. Once cool, peel and crush the garlic cloves, mix well with the yogurt and tahini and season with salt and pepper.

To make the herb topping, chop the pine nuts, parsley, mint and basil. De-seed the chilli, zest the lemon and finely chop the onion, zest and chilli. Combine well in a separate bowl.

Gently spread the dressing over the ocean trout, then press the herb topping evenly over the top of the fish.

Transfer to a serving plate. Top with rocket and drizzle with extra virgin olive oil.

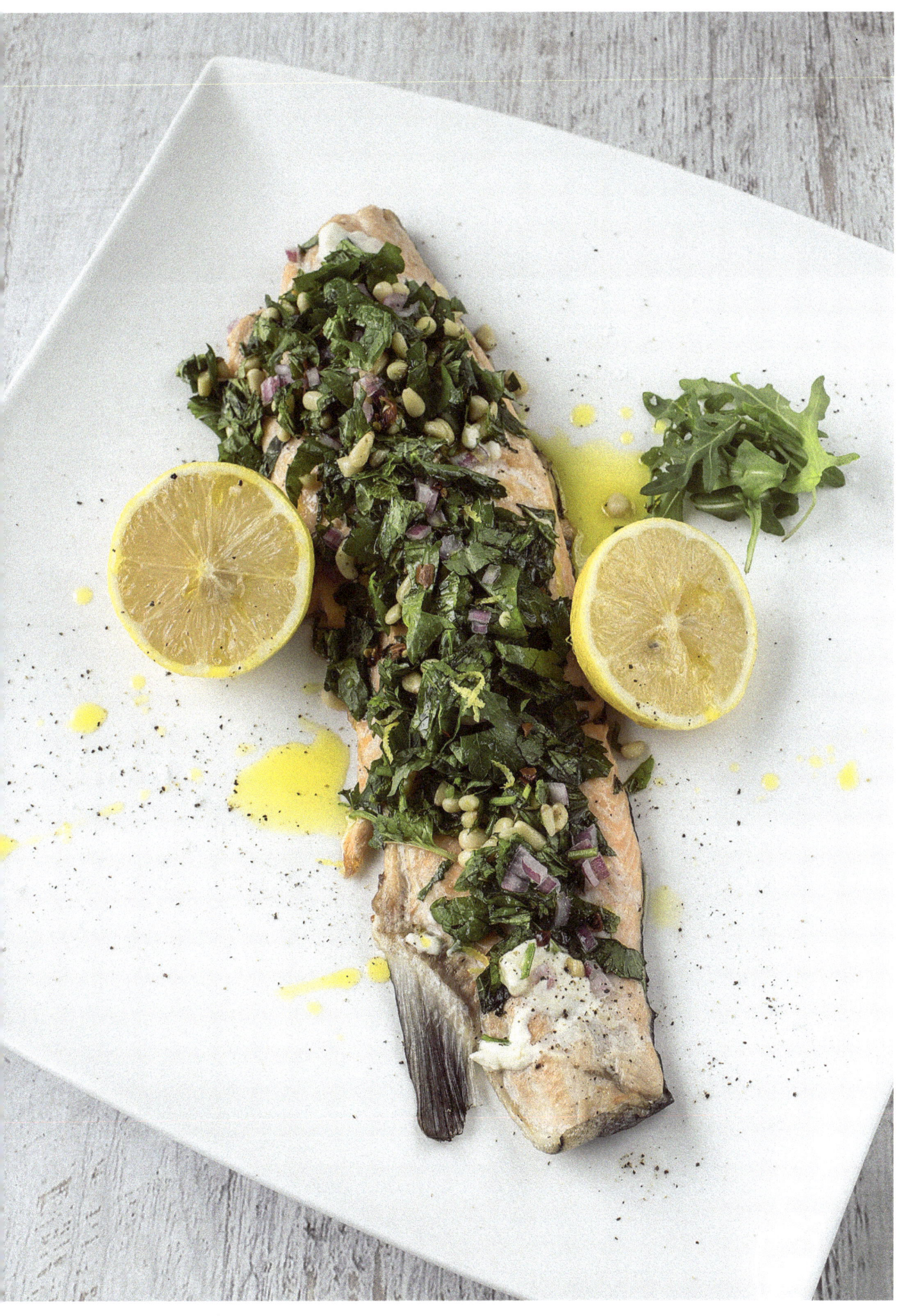

TASSAL

One Pot Salmon

SERVES 4

Chat potatoes are a small, floury potato. Substitute other floury varieties, chopped into large chunks. This dish will also work well with peeled and cubed pumpkin or sweet potato and diced red capsicum.

400 grams chat potatoes

4 fresh beetroot

4 garlic cloves

2 tablespoons extra virgin olive oil

1 bunch of fresh rosemary

2 lemons

8 asparagus spears

1 bunch broccolini

8 small vine tomatoes

4 x 180 gram Tassal salmon portions

1 tablespoon olive oil, to finish

¼ cup basil leaves

Preheat oven to 200°C.

Halve the potatoes, peel and chop the beetroot into 2cm cubes, peel the garlic and tip into an ovenproof casserole dish. Drizzle with extra virgin olive oil, sprinkle with rosemary, place into the oven and roast for 30 minutes, or until the vegetables are starting to brown.

Quarter the lemons. Remove the dish from the oven and add the asparagus spears, broccolini, tomatoes and lemons. Nestle the salmon amongst the vegetables. Return to the oven to cook for a further 10-15 minutes, until the salmon is cooked to your liking.

Remove from oven and drizzle with the remaining oil and garnish with basil leaves. Serve immediately, straight from the dish.

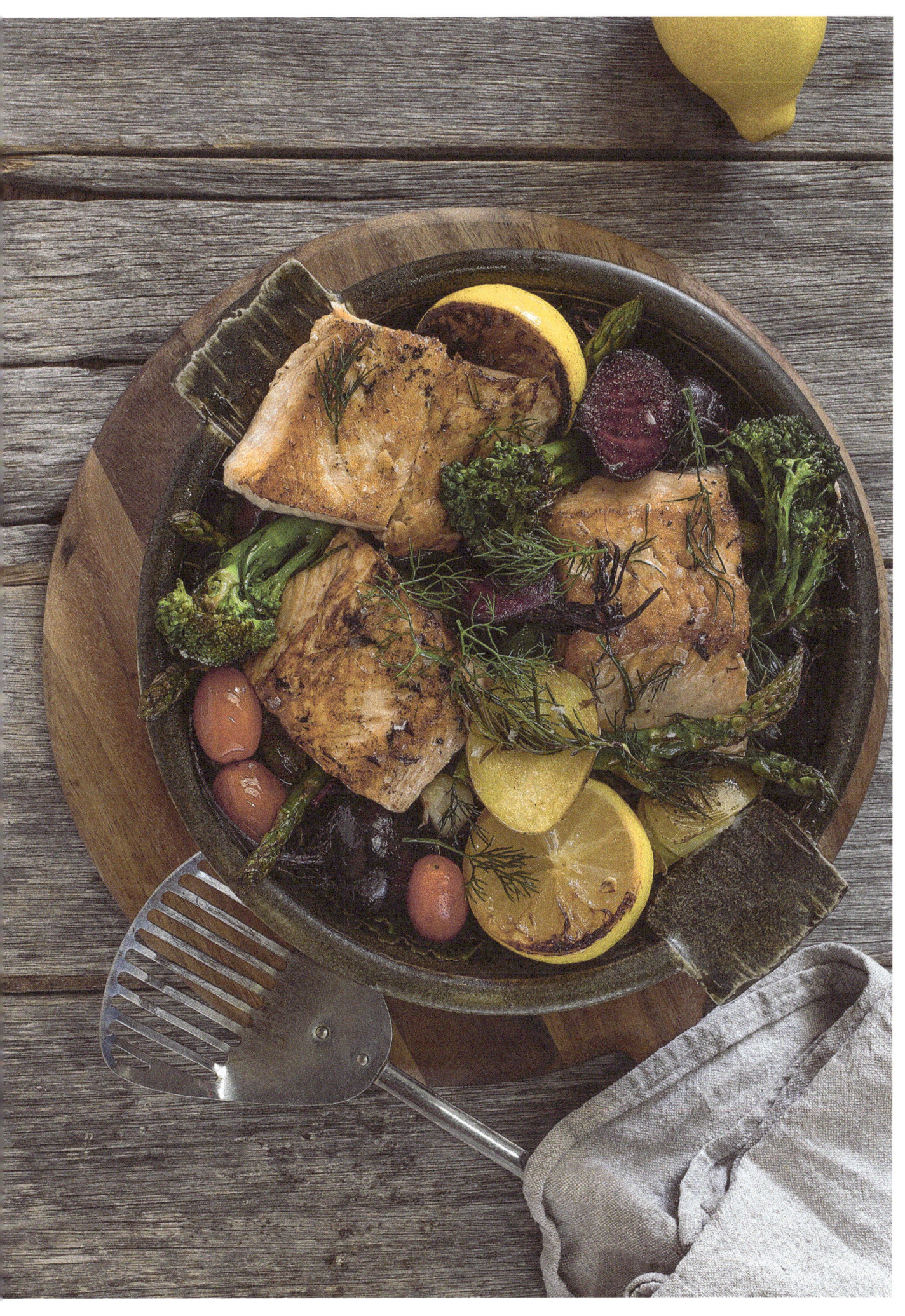

Buttermilk Blinis with Superior Gold Smoked Salmon

SERVES 12 AS A CANAPÉ

These blini are a fabulous canapé and also make a fancy breakfast! For a breakfast treat, simply increase the size of each blini – use 2 tablespoons of mixture, instead of one. Salmon pearls are the roe of the salmon – they look and taste beautiful as a garnish and are usually available at fishmongers and specialty fish shops such as the Tassal Salmon Shop.

200 grams creme fraiche

2 tablespoons horseradish puree

20 grams butter

1 cup plain flour

1 teaspoon caster sugar

2 teaspoons baking powder

1 teaspoon salt

1 tablespoon fresh dill

1 cup buttermilk

1 egg

200 grams Superior Gold smoked salmon

1 tablespoon chives

salmon pearls or caviar, to garnish

To make the horseradish cream, mix the creme fraiche and horseradish puree together in a small bowl, and set aside.

Melt the butter in the microwave in a small bowl, and set aside.

To make the blini batter, combine the flour, sugar, baking powder and salt in a large mixing bowl. Finely chop the dill and whisk into the flour mixture, along with the buttermilk and lightly beaten egg.

To cook the blini, heat a large frying pan over medium heat. Brush with melted butter. Spoon tablespoons of mixture into the pan, and cook for one minute on each side, until the blini are golden brown. Remove from the pan and repeat with the remaining batter, brushing melted butter onto the pan before cooking each batch.

Top each blini with pieces of smoked salmon, the horseradish cream, finely chopped chives and salmon pearls.

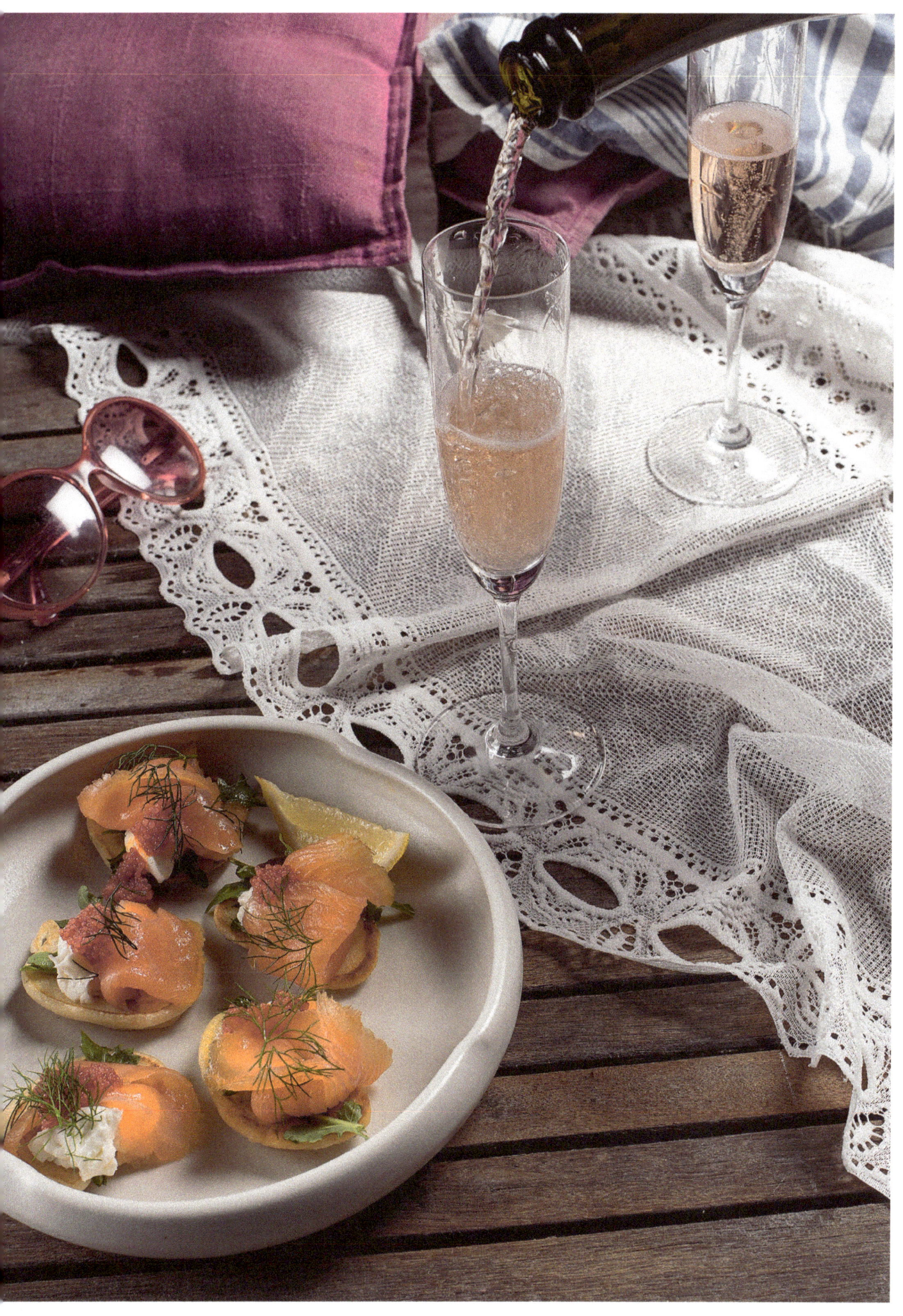

CHEXI - BROCKERLY ESTATE SPRING BAY SEAFOODS

Spring Bay Mussels A la Brava

SERVES 4

When tomatoes are in season in Tasmania, it's well worth making your own tomato sauce. It tastes amazing, and any additional sauce can be frozen for a later use. Unopened mussels are fine to eat, despite the myth! Simply prise them open with a paring knife and enjoy. This classic dish is delicious served with crusty bread and a green salad.

TOMATO SAUCE

2 tablespoons extra virgin olive oil

300 grams fresh tomatoes

½ teaspoon raw sugar

pinch of salt

pinch or two of cayenne pepper (or to taste)

1 brown onion

1 fresh bay leaf

1 teaspoon smoked Spanish paprika

125ml Tasmanian white wine

½ bunch parsley to garnish

LEMON MAYONNAISE

1 egg

juice of ½ lemon

¼ teaspoon curry powder

pinch of salt

150ml light extra virgin olive oil

1 kilogram mussels

To make the tomato sauce, heat 1 tablespoon of the extra virgin olive oil in a large, heavy-based saucepan over medium heat. Add the whole tomatoes, sugar and a pinch of salt and cayenne pepper, and cook slowly for 10-15 minutes or until the tomatoes have broken down.

Remove from the heat and tip the tomato mixture into a colander resting over a large bowl. Press the mixture through a colander to remove the skins and seeds. Discard the skins and seeds and set the tomato puree aside. Heat 1 tablespoon of oil in a clean, large, heavy-based saucepan over low heat.

Dice the onion and add to the pan along with the bay leaf, and smoked paprika and cook gently for 10 minutes or until well softened. Add the white wine, bring to the boil and reduce by half. Add the pureed tomatoes to the saucepan and simmer for 8 minutes. Remove the bay leaf and blend the sauce using a stick mixer.

To make the lemon mayonnaise, use a blender or food processor to blend the egg, lemon juice, curry powder and a pinch of salt. With the motor running, slowly add the oil in a steady drizzle to create a thick and creamy emulsion.

To prepare the mussels, clean the mussel shells well and remove any beards. Bring a shallow frying pan of water to the boil over medium heat. Once the water is boiling, add the mussels and remove each one as it opens to avoid overcooking.

To serve, remove the empty shell half from each mussel. Arrange the mussels onto the serving plates. Top each mussel with tomato sauce and a spoonful of lemon mayonnaise. Finely chop the parsley and sprinkle on top. Forget the cutlery for these mussels and provide lots of napkins instead - simply pick up the shell with your fingers, slurp and enjoy!

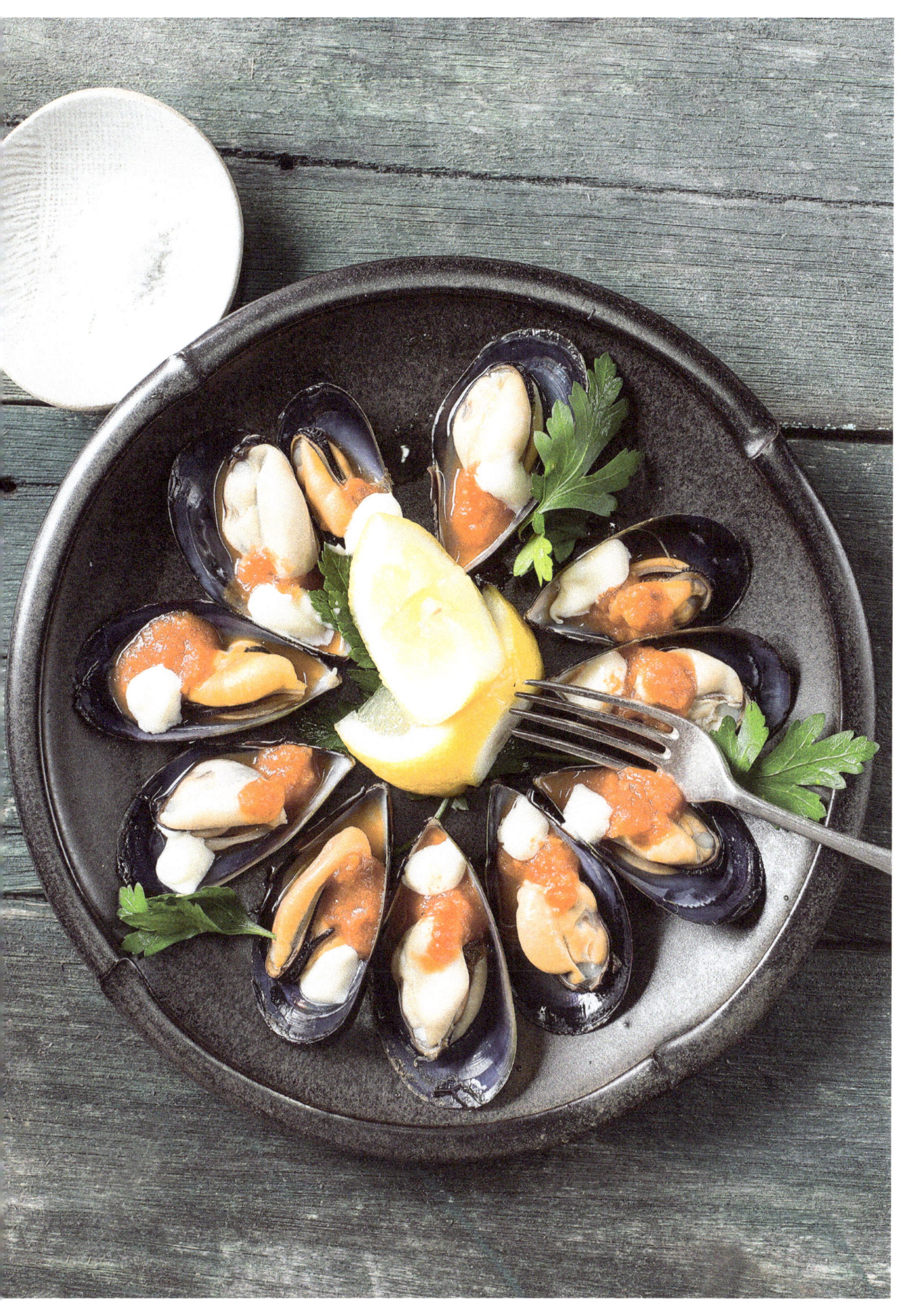

Lavender Salmon Gravlax with a Pickled Baby Beetroot, Radish and Snow Pea Salad and Garlic Croutons

SERVES 6 AS AN ENTRÉE OR LIGHT LUNCH

Gravlax is surprisingly easy to prepare and is so tasty. It makes a gorgeous celebration dish and I love to have it on my table for big family celebrations at Easter and Christmas. The lavender imparts a delicious scent and flavour that pairs well with the rich salmon.

SALMON GRAVLAX

30 grams Tasmanian pepper berries

20 grams dried juniper berries

20 grams lavender flowers

100 grams white sugar

2ml lavender essential oil

1 x 500 gram salmon fillet

30ml Tasmanian vodka

1 kilogram coarse rock salt

SALAD

1 bunch baby beetroot

50ml apple cider vinegar

50ml water

50 grams sugar

100 grams snow peas

1 bunch radishes

50 grams mixed microgreens

50 grams rocket

15ml extra virgin olive oil

CROUTONS

small sourdough baguette

100 grams butter

2 cloves garlic

To prepare the gravlax, place the pepper berries, juniper and lavender in a spice grinder and grind to a fine powder. Combine this pepper berry mixture with the sugar and lavender oil and spread over the salmon fillet. Spread a thin layer of rock salt over the base of a baking tray (just enough to cover the bottom). Place the salmon fillet on top of the salt, pour over the vodka, and then spread the remaining rock salt over the fillet. Place into the refrigerator to cure for 24 hours.

After 24 hours, remove the salmon fillet, brush off excess salt and rinse under cold running water to remove the last of the salt. Using a thin blade knife, slice the salmon into fine strips.

To prepare the salad, peel the beetroot and use a mandolin to slice them into 1mm slices. Cut the tops off the snow peas. Using a small saucepan, bring the vinegar, water and sugar to the boil over medium heat, add the sliced beetroot and set aside to cool. Drain once cooled. Bring a saucepan of salted water to the boil, drop in the snow peas and cook for 30 seconds. Drain immediately and refresh in iced water. Use the mandolin to slice the radishes into 1mm slices. Mix the beetroot, radish, snow peas, rocket and microgreens in a bowl with the olive oil.

To make the croutons, crush the garlic and place into saucepan with the butter. Slowly melt and bring to a simmer. Remove from the heat. Slice the sourdough into 5mm thick strips, brush with the garlic butter mixture and bake at 160°C for 12 minutes, or until crisp and golden brown. Leave to cool.

Serve the sliced salmon with the salad and garlic croutons.

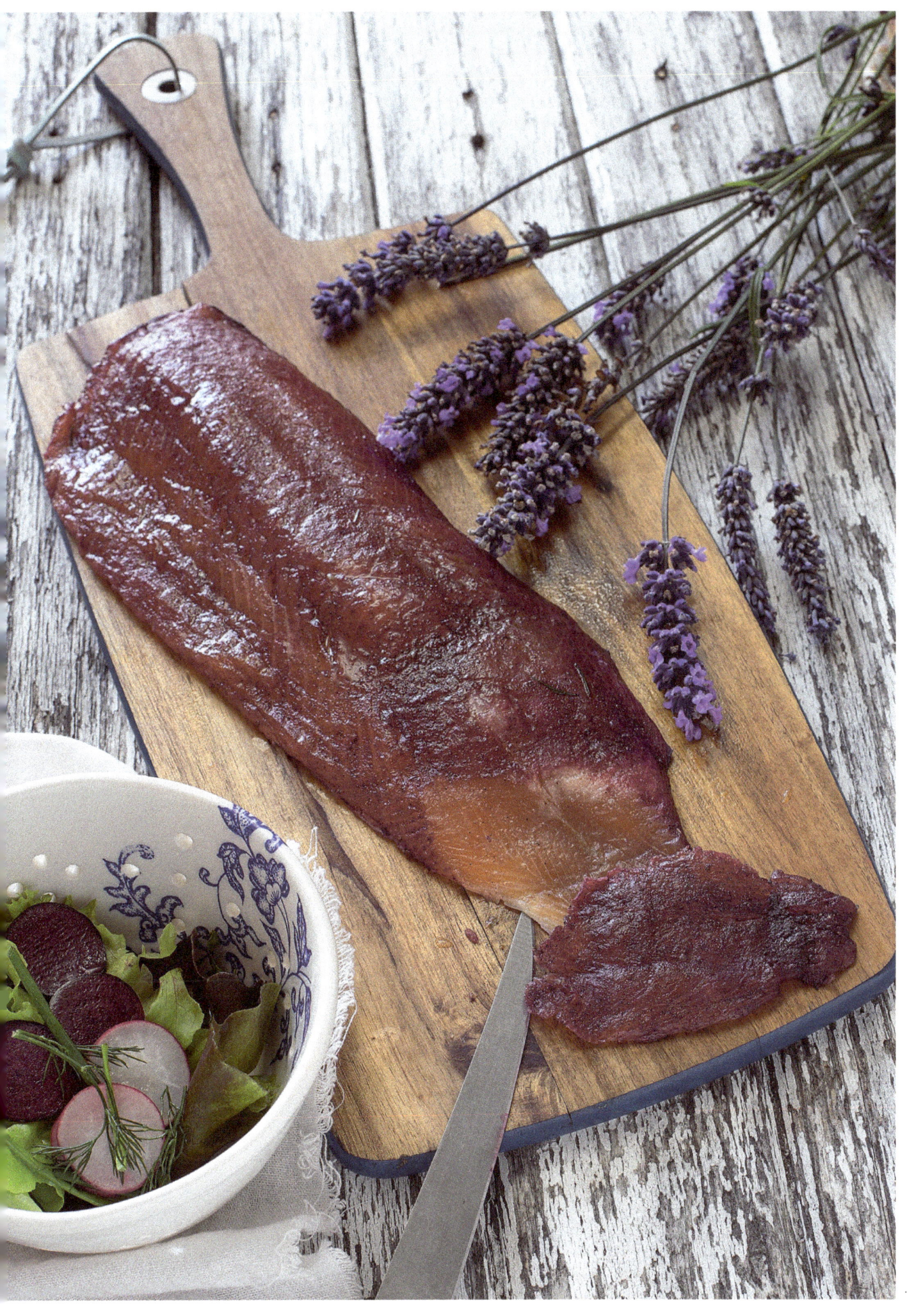

HUON AQUACULTURE

Red Miso Huon Salmon

SERVES 4

3 limes or lemons

½ cup red miso paste

2 tablespoons rice bran oil

4 x 140 gram Huon Aquaculture salmon portions

1 cup baby corn

2 cups pre-cooked hokkien noodles

2 bunches bok choy

To prepare the marinade, juice 2 lemons or limes and combine the juice with the red miso paste. Coat the salmon liberally with the marinade.

Using a large frying pan, heat the rice bran oil over medium heat and place each salmon portion carefully into the pan. Cook for 1-2 minutes, then turn carefully. Add the baby corn, hokkien noodles and bok choy to the pan. Cook for a further 5-6 minutes until the bok choy is wilted and the Huon Salmon is cooked through.

Place the Huon Salmon portions on each plate on a bed of the noodles, baby corn and bok choy. Cut the remaining lemon or lime into wedges and serve with the salmon and noodles.

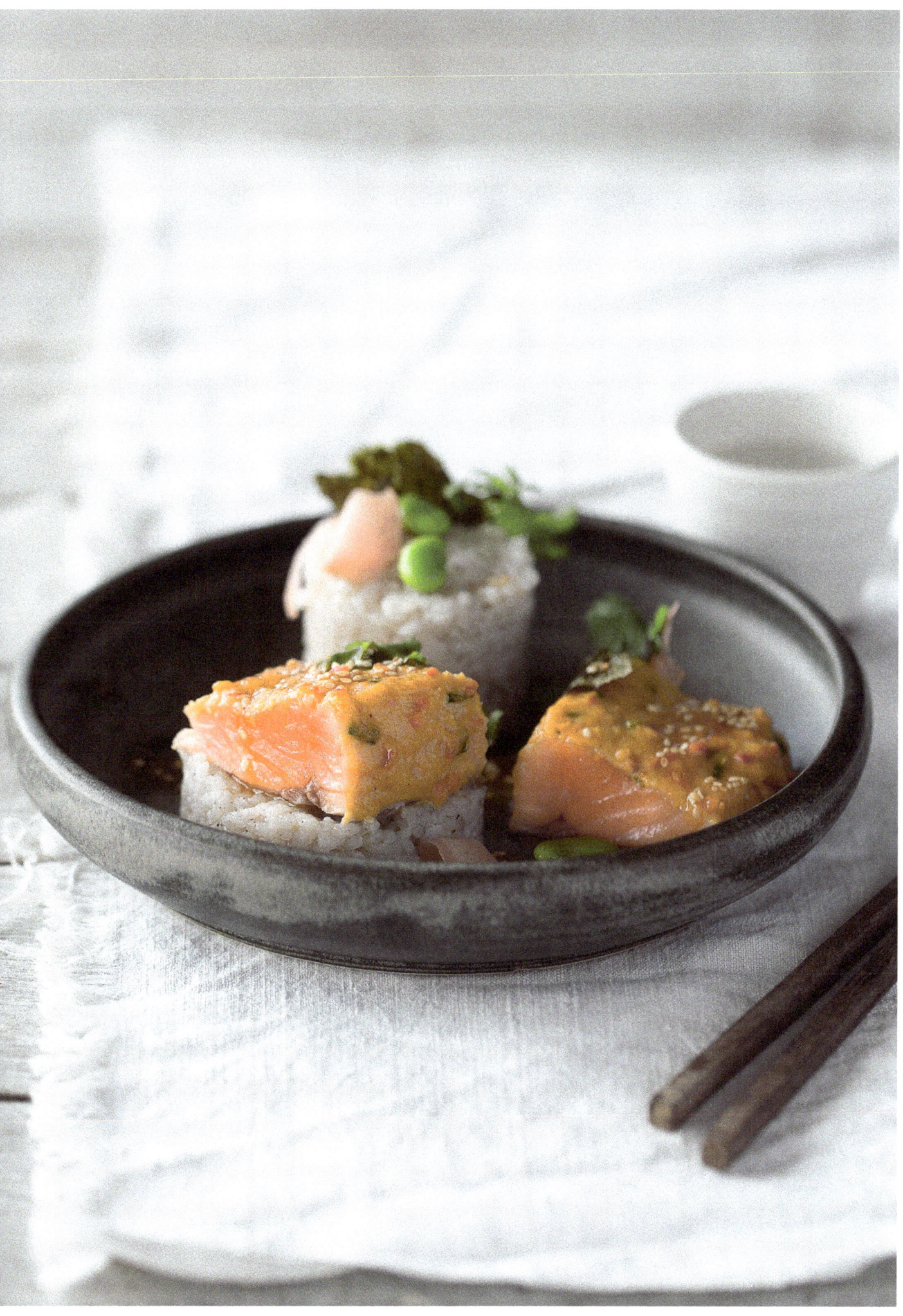

HUON AQUACULTURE

Huon Wood Roasted Salmon Frittata

SERVES 4

1 red or yellow capsicum

1 cup sweet potato

6 large free range eggs

½ cup cream

2 cups baby spinach

1 x 150 gram Huon Aquaculture Wood Roasted hot smoked salmon

salt and pepper

1 tablespoon olive oil

Preheat the oven to 180°C.

Thinly slice the capsicum and sweet potato and combine in a large bowl, along with the eggs, cream and baby spinach, and season with salt and pepper.

Heat the oil in a large, non-stick frying pan over medium to low heat. Carefully pour in the egg mixture and top with flaked pieces of salmon. Cook for 3 minutes.

Remove from the heat and cook in the oven for 20 minutes, or until the frittata is firm and golden brown on top.

Serve with bread and salad for a more substantial meal.

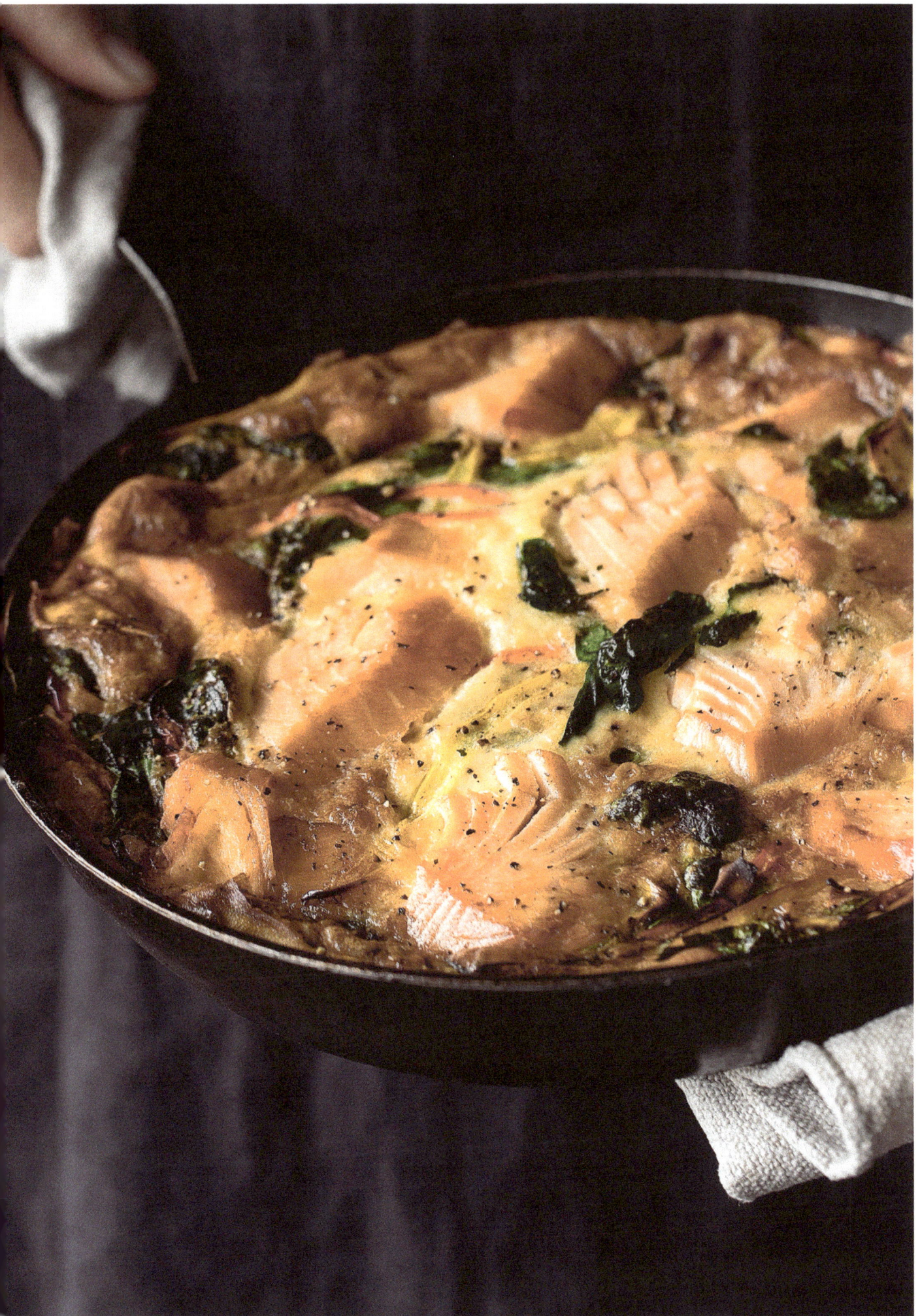

Summer Vegetable and Salmon Pasta

SERVES 4

My entire family loves this quick pasta - it's filled with delicious veggies, which is always a bonus when you're feeding children! Smoked salmon offcuts or canned salmon would be suitable in to use in this recipe, there's no need to buy premium grade salmon. Making your own pasta is easy and fun, but using a packet of pasta is a very quick alternative – simply cook according to packet instructions and add to the hot sauce before serving.

PASTA

200 grams plain flour

1 tablespoon oil

2 eggs

SAUCE

1 tablespoon extra virgin olive oil

3 large cloves garlic

1 red onion

1 zucchini

2 yellow squash

300 grams snow peas

1 punnet cherry tomatoes

100 grams spinach

½ bunch dill

½ bunch parsley

400 grams smoked salmon

2 tablespoons sundried tomatoes

80 grams Parmesan cheese

sea salt and cracked pepper

Use a food processor to make the pasta dough. Tip the flour into the processor, turn on and add the oil and the eggs with the motor running. Continue blending until the mixture comes together to form a firm dough. If the mixture seems too wet or sticky to handle, knead in a little more flour by hand on a floured bench.

To roll the pasta, divide the dough into 4 portions. Using a pasta machine set at number 1 (or at the widest setting) feed each portion of the dough through the machine. Repeat this process with each portion of pasta on each setting, until you reach setting number 6, (or the narrowest setting on your machine). The pasta should be silky smooth and slightly elastic. Cut the pasta into fettuccini strips using the appropriate cutter on the pasta machine. Dust the bench with flour and carefully lay the pasta aside until needed.

To cook the fettuccini, bring a large saucepan of salted water to the boil and cook the fettuccini for 4 minutes. Alternatively, the pasta can be cooked in advance, even the day before it is required. To do so, simply cook the fettuccini as above, cool and roll in a little olive oil and refrigerate until required. Reheat the fettuccini in the sauce when you are ready to serve the dish.

To make the pasta sauce, heat the oil in a heavy-based frying pan over medium heat. Crush the garlic, slice the onion and sauté for 3 minutes, or until the onion has softened. Slice the zucchini and squash, add the pan and continue to cook, stirring occasionally, for 3 minutes or until the vegetables are soft. Remove the ends from the snow peas and halve, halve the cherry tomatoes and roughly chop the spinach, dill and parsley. Reduce the heat to low, and add the snow peas, tomatoes, spinach, dill and parsley and continue to cook until the spinach and herbs are just wilted. Remove from the heat and toss the hot pasta, salmon and sundried tomatoes through the sauce. To serve, top with grated or shaved Parmesan cheese and season well with salt and pepper.

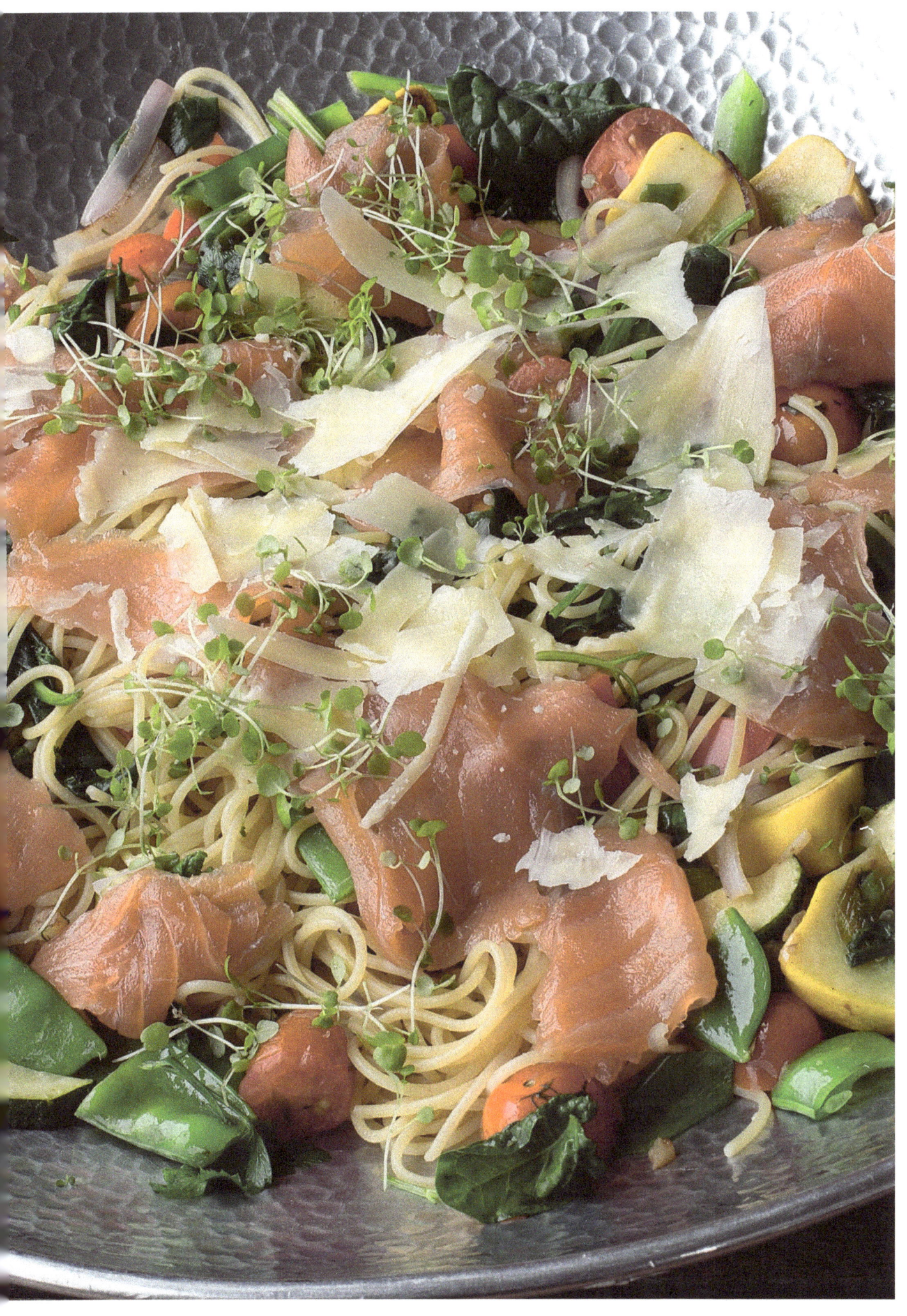

Spring Bay Mussels in a Tomato and Tarragon Broth with Saffron Aioli

SERVES 4

Making your own fish broth makes all the difference to the flavour of this dish. After cooking, it does need to stand for a few hours for the flavours to fully develop, so get the broth started earlier in the day if you are planning this dish for dinner. You can keep fish bones and skin or prawn shells from other recipes, store them into a ziplock bag in the freezer and then use them for the broth when you're ready.

BROTH

1 tablespoon olive oil

1 onion

1 clove garlic

½ teaspoon fennel seed

1 tablespoon dried tarragon

500 grams tomatoes

250 grams fish bones, skin and/or prawn shells

1 ½ tablespoons tomato paste

¼ cup plain flour

½ cup lemon juice

125ml cup white wine

2 litres water

salt and pepper

SAFFRON AIOLI

2 egg yolks

1 egg

30ml white vinegar

¼ teaspoon saffron threads

1 clove garlic

salt and pepper

200ml light olive oil

1 kilogram black Spring Bay mussels

1 cup spinach leaves

1 small baguette

To make the stock, heat the oil in a large saucepan over medium heat. Roughly chop the onion, finely chop the garlic and add to the pot along with the fennel seeds and tarragon, and cook for 3 minutes or until the onion is softened. Add the tomatoes, fish bones, tomato paste and flour and cook for a further 3 minutes.

Add the lemon juice, wine and water, bring to the boil, reduce the heat and simmer for 25 minutes. Remove from the heat, season with salt and pepper and set aside for a few hours for the flavours to develop before straining through a sieve.

To make the aioli, use a blender or food processor to combine the egg yolks, whole egg, vinegar, saffron, garlic and a sprinkle of salt and pepper. With the motor running, slowly add the oil in a steady drizzle to create a thick, creamy emulsion.

To cook the mussels, clean and de-beard each mussel and shred the spinach. Bring the broth to the boil, add the mussels and cook for a few minutes, or until they open.

Stir through the shredded spinach and serve immediately with sliced baguette for soaking up the delicious juices, and the saffron aioli.

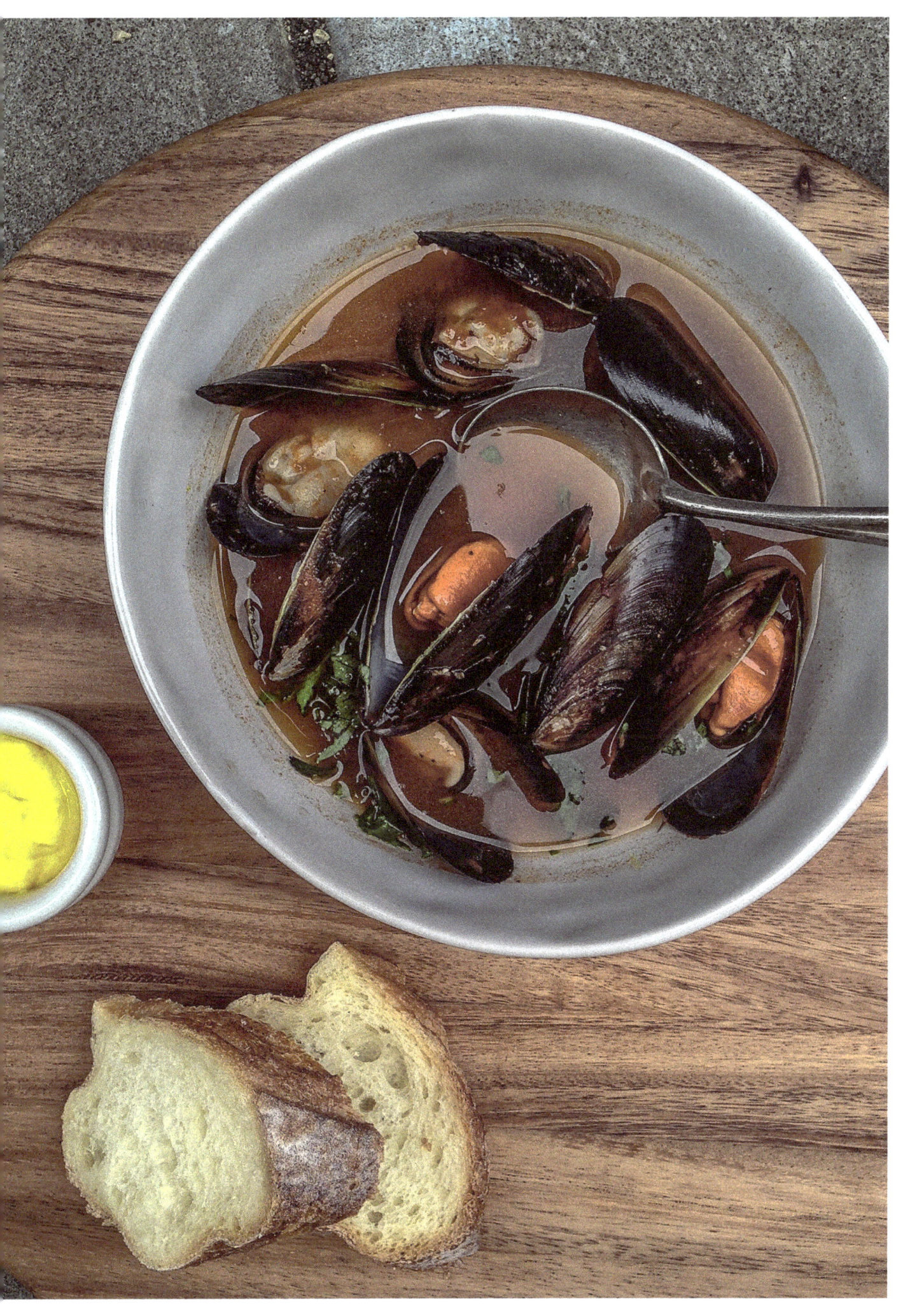

GET SHUCKED - BRUNY ISLAND OYSTERS

Steamy Oriental Oysters

MAKES 12

1cm piece of ginger

1 long red chilli

1 spring onion

1 heaped teaspoon white miso paste

juice of 1 lime

3 teaspoons sugar

300ml hot water

12 Get Shucked Bruny Island Pacific Oysters

Peel and grate the ginger, de-seed and finely chop the chilli and finely chop the spring onion. Combine in a small bowl along with the miso paste, lime juice, sugar and hot water, and stir until the miso paste and sugar have dissolved.

Bring a saucepan of water to the boil, lay the oysters into a bamboo steamer and place the steamer on top of the saucepan. Spoon the oriental broth over the oysters. Cover with the lid and steam the oysters for 10 minutes until they are cooked through.

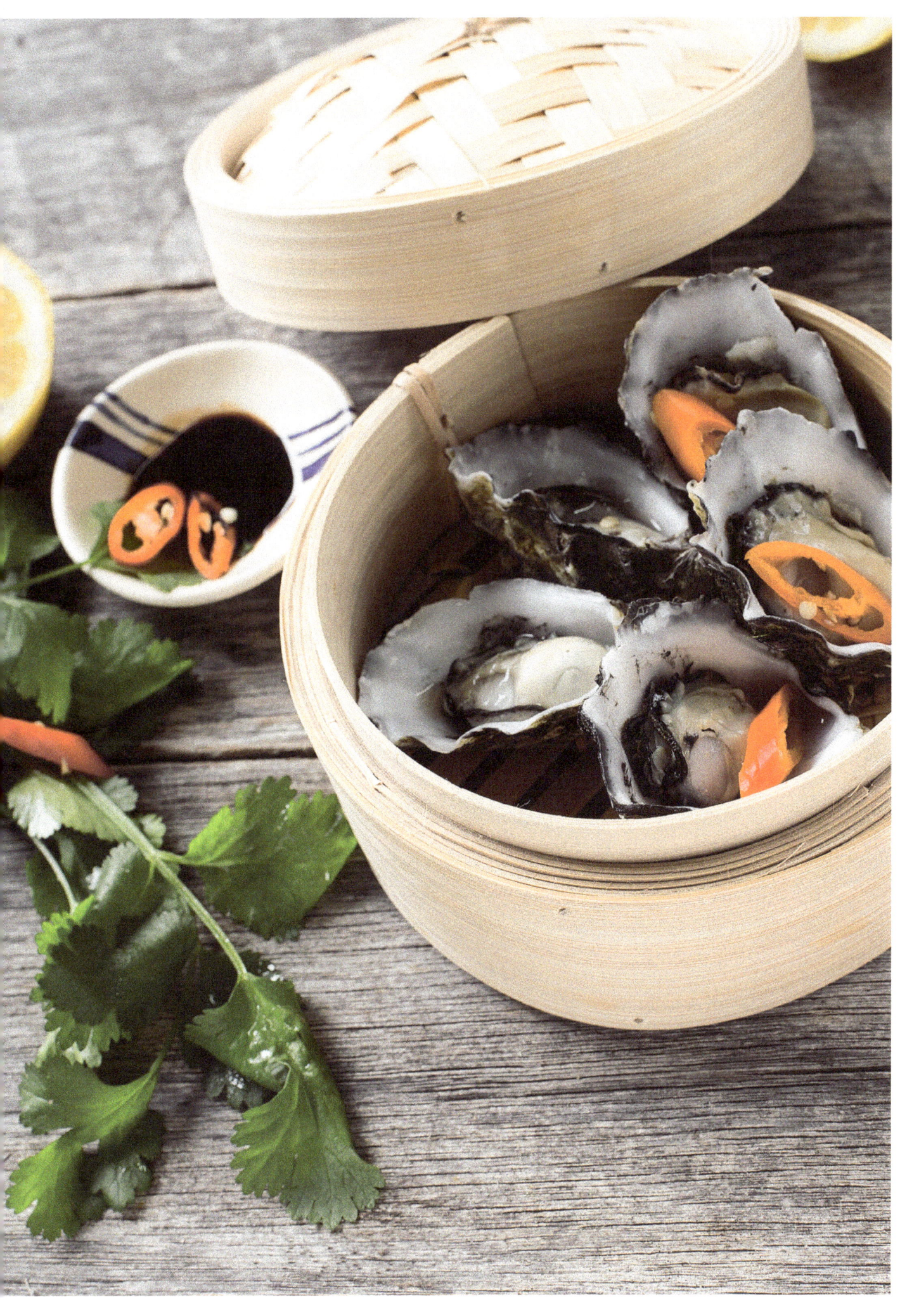

Crispy Pepper Berry Tassal Salmon with Ashbolt Sparkling Elderflower

SERVES 2

This elegant yet super-simple dish takes just 10 minutes to prepare and another 10 to minutes to cook. Ashbolt Elderflower Sparkling has a delicate flavour of ginger, lychees, flowers and lemons, and elder has been used historically as a de-tox – it is a wonderful non-alcoholic alternative to sparkling wine.

4-5 dried pepper berries

1 tablespoon sea salt

2 x 200-250 gram Tassal salmon portions

30ml extra virgin olive oil

1 x 330ml bottle Ashbolt Elderflower Sparkling

1 bunch asparagus

3 baby leeks

50 grams cold unsalted butter

1 punnet micro lemon balm

salt & pepper

Using a mortar and pestle, make a pepper berry salt by grinding the pepper berries and sea salt together. Rub this salt over the skin of each salmon portion.

Heat the oil in a frying pan over medium heat and wait until the oil starts to smoke (this will take around 30-40 seconds). Place salmon into the frying pan, skin side down, and cook for 2-3 minutes. Carefully turn the salmon and pour in sparkling elderflower. Cook for a further 2-3 minutes. The sparkling elderflower will reduce and create the base of the sauce.

Slice the asparagus and leeks, add to the pan and cook for 1-2 minutes. Remove the salmon and vegetables from the pan and arrange on plates. Whisk the cubed butter into the pan, 10 grams at a time, until the sauce has thickened.

Garnish with the micro lemon balm, season to taste and serve.

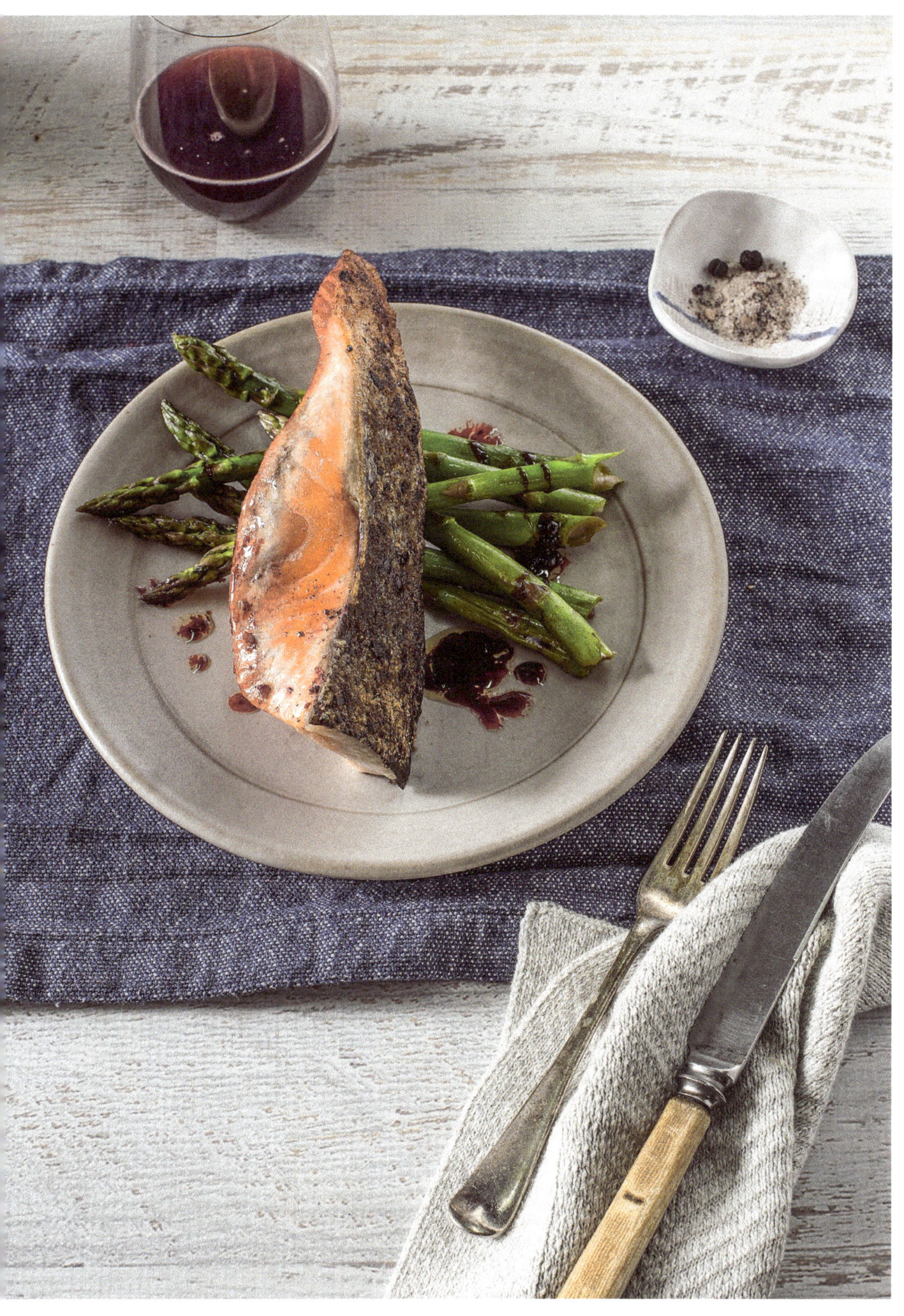

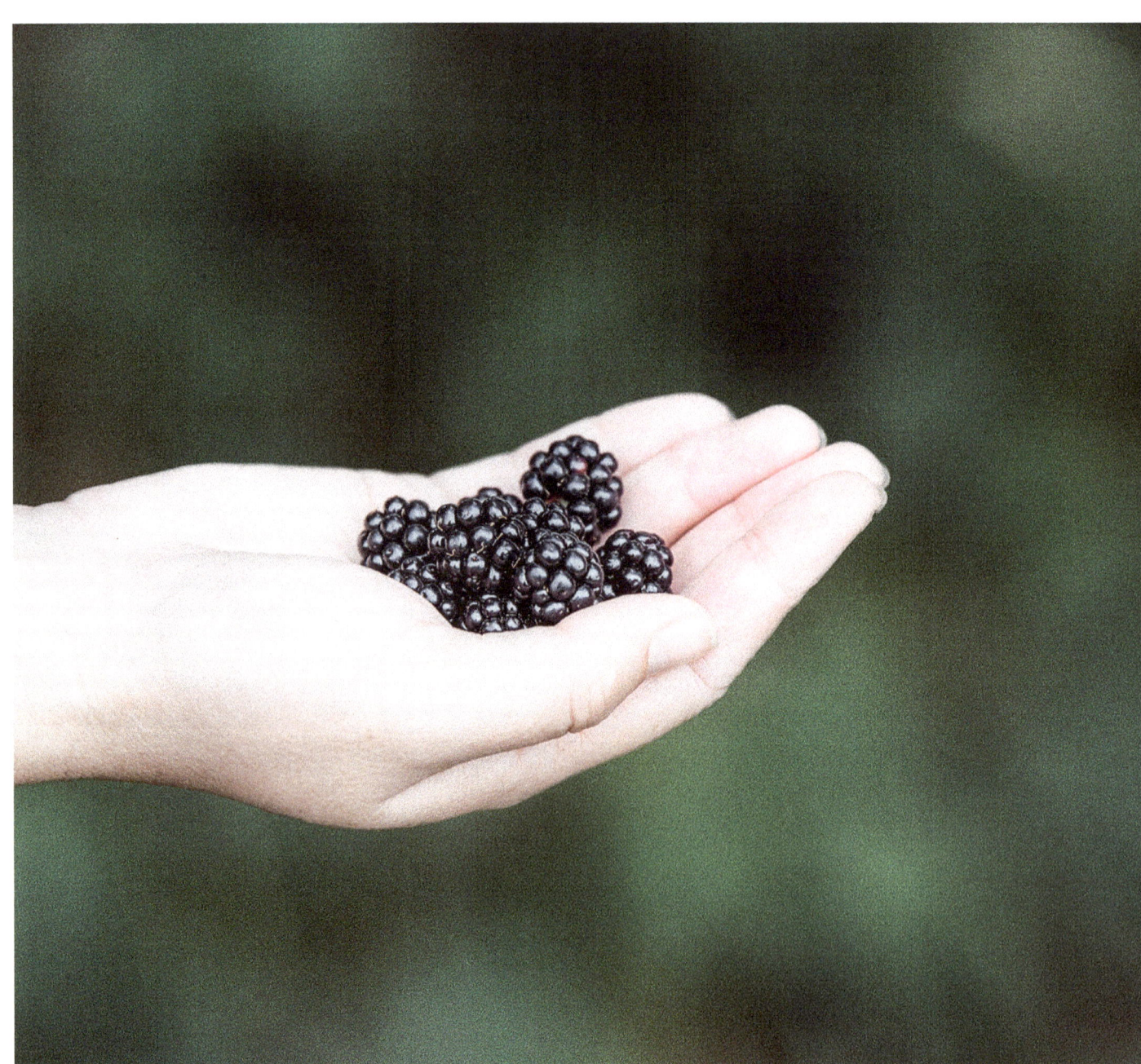

From the Wild

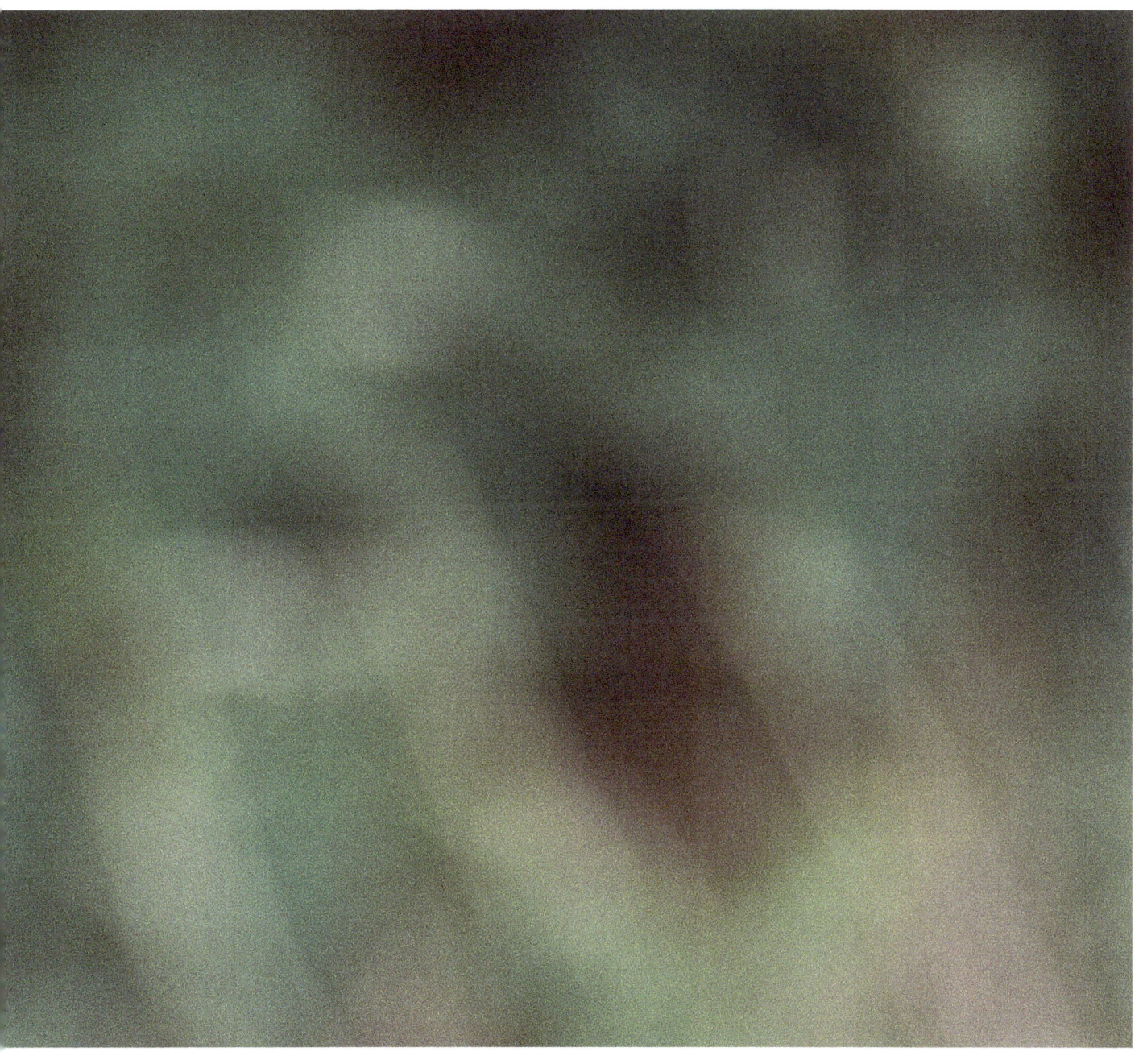

Slow Cooked Rabbit with Fresh Pasta

SERVES 4

Rabbit has a delicious, subtle gamey flavour and this dish is delicious served over hot pasta.

PASTA

200 grams plain flour

1 tablespoon oil

2 eggs

SAUCE

2 brown onions

3 cloves garlic

1 whole rabbit

400 grams chopped tomatoes

2 tablespoons basil

2 tablespoons oregano

2 tablespoons parsley

250ml white wine

200ml cream

80 grams Parmesan cheese

Use a food processor to make the pasta dough. Tip the flour into the processor, turn on and add the oil and the eggs with the motor running. Continue blending until the mixture comes together to form a firm dough. If the mixture seems too wet or sticky to handle, knead in a little more flour by hand on a floured bench.

To roll the pasta, divide the dough into 4 portions. Using a pasta machine set at number 1 (or at the widest setting) feed each portion of the dough through the machine. Repeat this process with each portion of pasta on each setting, until you reach setting number 6, (or the narrowest setting on your machine). The pasta should be silky smooth and slightly elastic. Cut the pasta into fettuccini strips using the appropriate cutter on the pasta machine. Dust the bench with flour and carefully lay the pasta aside until needed.

To cook the fettuccini, bring a large saucepan of salted water to the boil and cook the fettuccini for 4 minutes. Alternatively, the pasta can be cooked in advance, even the day before it is required. To do so, simply cook the fettuccini as above, cool and roll in a little olive oil and refrigerate until required. Reheat the fettuccini in the sauce when you are ready to serve the dish.

Finely dice the onion, crush the garlic and tip into the bottom of a slow cooker, or into a braising pan if you are using the oven. Add the rabbit, tomatoes, herbs and wine. Cover and leave to cook in the slow cooker for 4-6 hours (depending on your slow cooker). If you are using the oven, cover the pan and cook for 2-3 hours at 160°C. When cooked, set aside to cool and remove all of the bones from the rabbit.

To create the sauce, tip the rabbit meat and liquid from the slow cooking into a heavy-based saucepan, add the cream, season well with salt and pepper and bring to a simmer over low heat. Cook until the sauce has thickened, but take care not to overcook or the sauce will split. Season well with sea salt and cracked pepper. Toss through the hot pasta and top with Parmesan cheese.

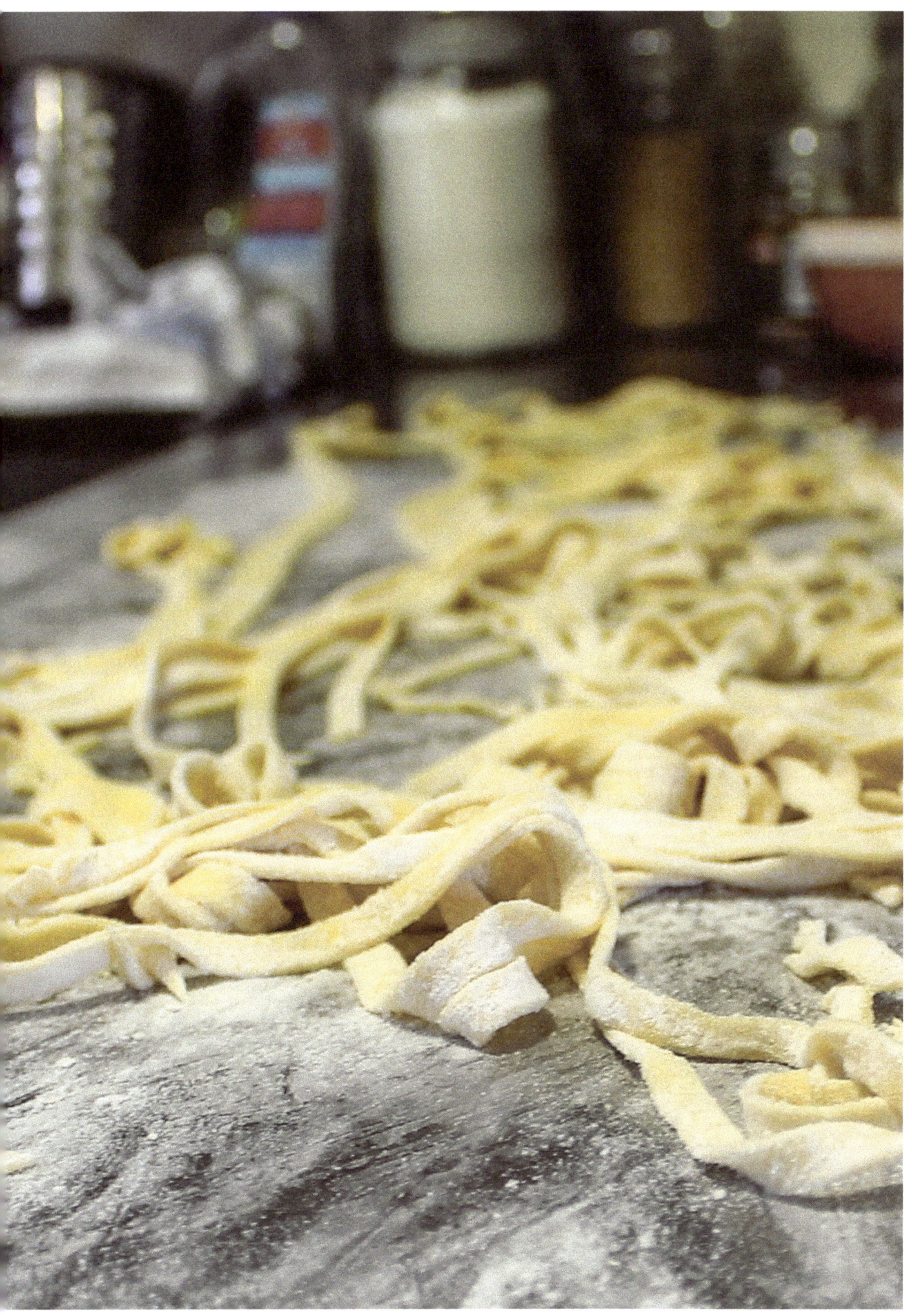

Grilled Wallaby with a Roast Beetroot, Roast Garlic and Goats Cheese Tart

SERVES 4

Pre-baking this tart makes this an easy and delicious dish to serve for a special dinner. To speed up the process, you can use 2 sheets of frozen shortcrust pastry, instead of making your own. The tart is also a delicious accompaniment to beef, chicken or lamb, or served on its own with quince paste and a fresh, green salad. To make your own quince paste, see the recipe on page 100.

TART FILLING

2 medium beetroot

2 bulbs garlic

1 tablespoon olive oil

1 tablespoon onion

1 tablespoon basil leaves

100 grams Tongola goat cheese

2 tablespoons Parmesan cheese

6 eggs

¾ cup cream

TART BASE

125 grams butter

1 ⅔ cups plain flour

1 tablespoon water

4 x 150 gram wallaby fillets

extra virgin olive oil to coat

Preheat the oven to 180°C. Grease a 20cm pie dish or tart tin.

To cook the vegetables for the tart, dice the beetroot into 1cm cubes and peel the garlic cloves. Tip beetroot and garlic into a baking tray, drizzle over oil to coat and roast in the oven for 18 minutes, or until soft and cooked through. Set aside to cool.

Meanwhile, use a food processor to make the pastry. Cut the butter into cubes, tip the flour into the processor, add the butter and pulse until the mixture resembles fine crumbs. With the motor running, add the water and process until the mixture comes forms a smooth dough – you may need to add a little extra water to help the mixture come together. Knead well on a floured bench, wrap in plastic wrap and set aside to rest for half an hour. Roll the pastry out to 5mm thick use to line the pie dish.

To make the tart filling, dice the onion and shred the basil leaves, grate or chop the goat cheese and grate the Parmesan. In a large bowl, whisk together the eggs and cream until well combined, then stir through the onion, basil, cheeses, beetroot and garlic and mix well. Pour the filling into the tart base. Bake in the oven for 18 minutes, or until golden brown and set.

To cook the wallaby fillets, coat each fillet with a little olive oil and pan fry or grill over medium-high heat for 8 minutes. This will cook the wallaby to medium-rare – adjust the cooking time to suit your preferences. Set aside to rest wrapped in foil after cooking.

To serve, slice the wallaby fillet, and arrange on a plate with a slice of tart and some homemade quince paste.

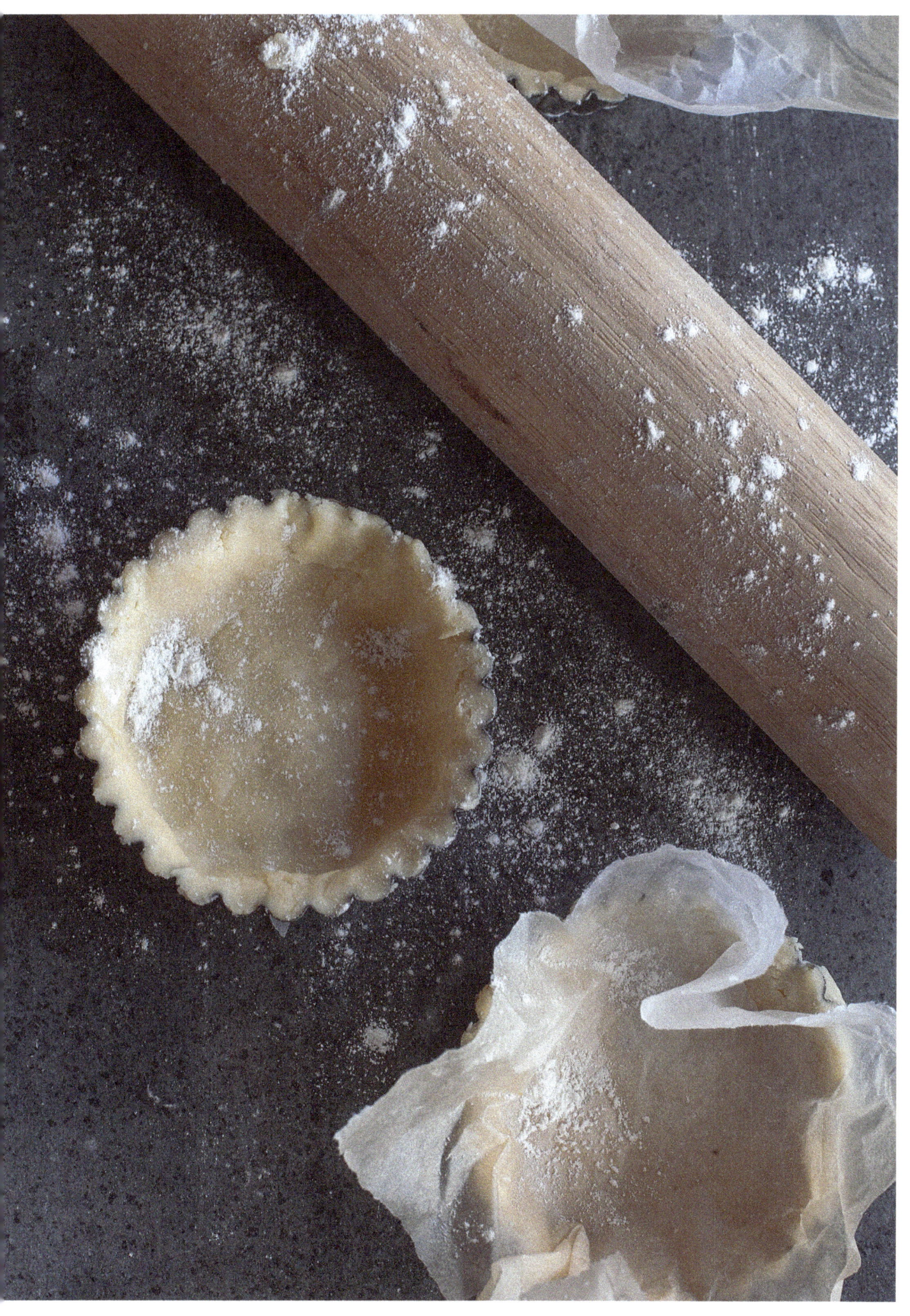

Seared Doo Town Wallaby with Beetroot Puree, Goat Cheese, and Spiced Balsamic Reduction

SERVES 4

1 tablespoon smoked paprika

1 tablespoon ground cumin

extra virgin olive oil

1 x 400 gram Doo Town wallaby fillet

200 grams whole beetroot

½ cup balsamic vinegar

1 tablespoon cumin

¼ cup brown sugar

salt and pepper

1 lemon

60 gram Tongola Zoe goat cheese (or a goat chevre)

100 grams rocket leaves

To prepare the wallaby, mix together the paprika and cumin with enough olive oil to make a paste, and rub this spice mix all over the wallaby fillet. Wrap well in plastic wrap and marinate in the refrigerator for 2- 6 hours.

To cook the vegetables, preheat the oven to 160°C and put the whole beetroots in a baking dish. Mix together the balsamic vinegar, cumin, brown sugar, and few grinds of salt and pepper in a small bowl, and pour over the beetroot. Pour enough water into the baking dish to come halfway up the beetroot. Cover with a tightly fitting lid, or with foil. Roast for 2 hours, or until the beetroot is tender, then set aside to cool slightly.

Pour the balsamic liquid from the baking dish into a heavy-based saucepan, and simmer over medium heat until the liquid has reduced by half, to create a beetroot reduction. Meanwhile, peel the beetroots by scraping the skin off with a paring knife, and cut into rough chunks. Place the beetroot into a food processor with 1 tablespoon of the balsamic reduction and the juice of half a lemon. Process the beetroots to a smooth puree. Taste for seasoning and adjust with salt, pepper, sugar and/or additional lemon juice as required – the puree should have an earthy, sweet flavour with a bit of zing from the lemon.

To cook the wallaby, heat a heavy griddle pan or flat frying pan over medium high heat. When the pan is hot, sear the wallaby on all sides for approximately one minute each side, depending on the thickness of the wallaby continue cooking until it is cooked to your liking. Remove from the heat and let the wallaby rest.

To serve, spread a portion of the beetroot puree on each place, slice the wallaby and arrange on top of the puree. Crumble or chop the goat cheese and sprinkle on top of the wallaby. Add rocket leaves on the side and drizzle with the balsamic reduction.

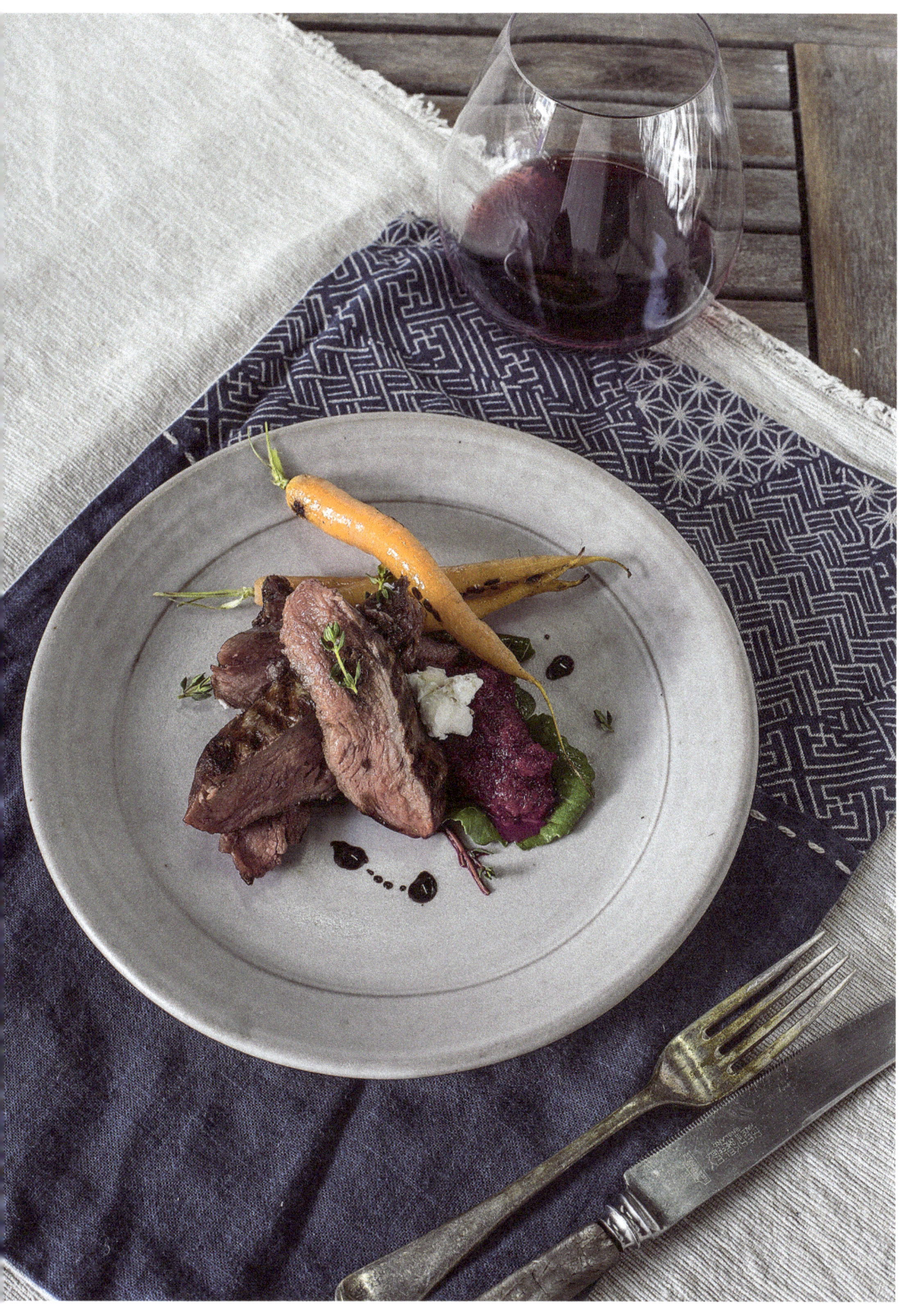

MEL COPPING - FELON'S BISTRO PORT ARTHUR HISTORIC SITE

Wallaby Ragout

SERVES 4-6

To make your own fresh pasta to accompany this hearty wallaby ragout, see the recipe on page 158

RAGOUT

1 onion

1 carrot

1 stick celery

4 cloves garlic

20 grams butter

2 chorizo sausages

500 grams wallaby mince

800 grams tomatoes

4 tablespoons parsley

4 tablespoons oregano

2 tablespoons tomato paste

salt and pepper

200 grams fresh pasta

1 tablespoon butter

80 grams Parmesan cheese

2 tablespoons parsley

To make the ragout, finely dice the onion, carrot and celery and crush the garlic. Melt the butter in a frying pan over medium heat, add the diced vegetables and sauté for 3 minutes, or until softened. Slice the chorizo and add to the frying pan along with the wallaby mince and cook, stirring, for 5 minutes or until the wallaby mince is well browned. Chop the tomatoes and herbs and add to the pan with the tomato paste, then continue to cook gently for 30 minutes. Season well with salt and pepper.

To cook the pasta, bring a large saucepan of water to the boil, drop in the pasta and cook for approximately 5 minutes, or until tender and al dente. Drain and stir through the butter.

Serve the hot, buttered pasta with the wallaby ragout, and top with shaved Parmesan cheese and finely chopped parsley.

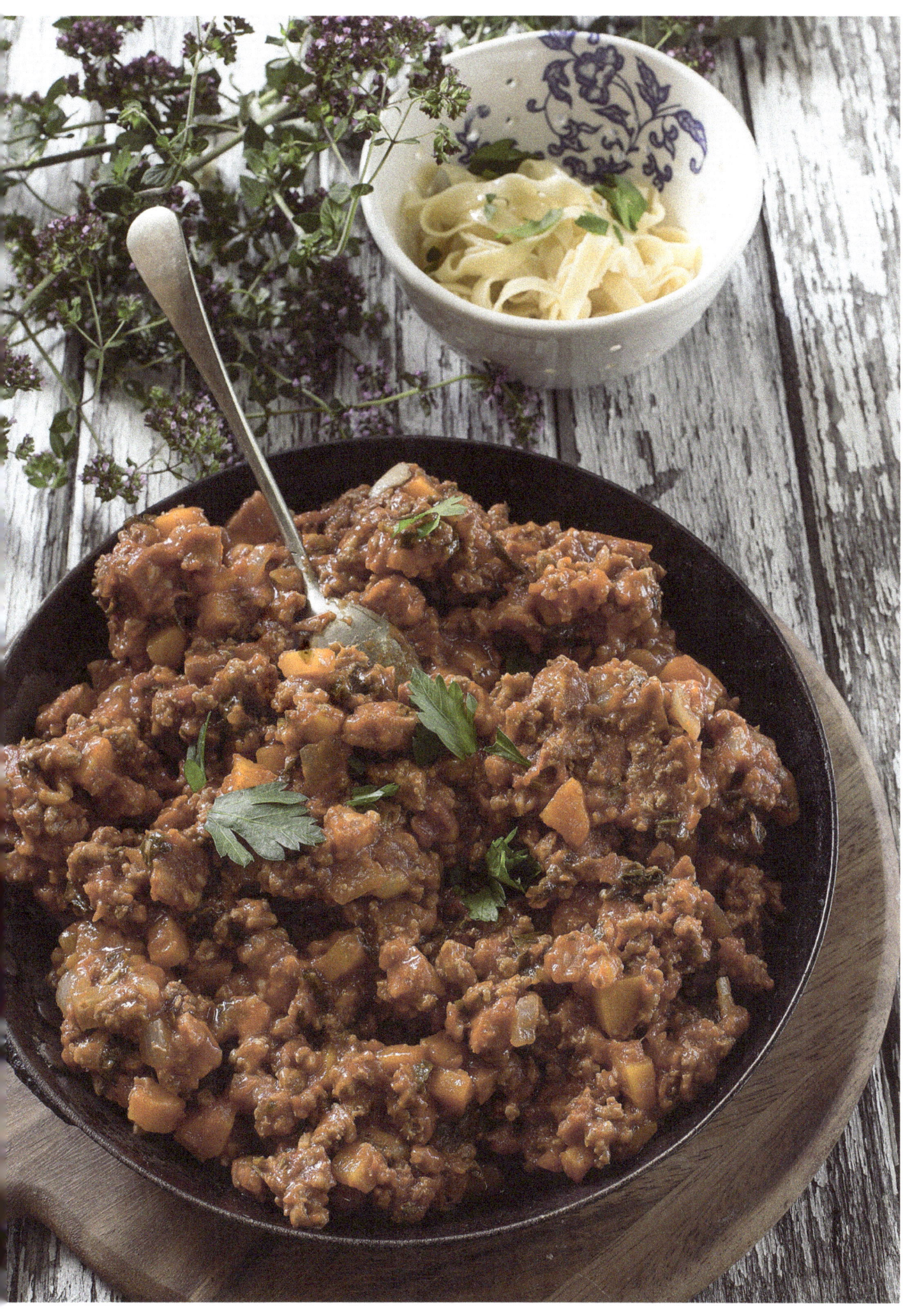

Wallaby Fillet with Thyme Roasted Beetroot, Feta and Cherry Chutney

SERVES 4

This spiced wallaby fillet is lovely served with a crisp green salad, or with mashed potatoes and vegetables.

CHERRY CHUTNEY

200 grams cherries

1 small red onion

2 tablespoons red wine vinegar

2 tablespoons brown sugar

WALLABY

2 large beetroot

5 sprigs thyme

1 tablespoon oil

1 cup silver-beet or spinach leaves

1 tablespoon black peppercorns

1 tablespoon pepper berries

4 x 150 gram wallaby fillets

1 teaspoon oil

120 grams feta cheese

To make the chutney, halve and stone the cherries and dice the onion. Put the cherries, onion, vinegar and brown sugar into a small saucepan and cook over low heat for half an hour, or until the cherries are soft and cooked through.

Preheat the oven to 180°C. Peel and dice the beetroot, and finely chop the thyme. Tip into a baking tray, drizzle with oil and bake for about 30 minutes, or until the beetroot are tender. Whilst the tray is still hot, toss through the silver beet or spinach and crumbled feta cheese.

To cook the wallaby, crush the peppercorns and pepper berries in a mortar and pestle and roll the wallaby fillets in this mixture to coat. Brush the fillets with oil, then heat a frying pan, grill or barbecue over high heat and cook for approximately 8 minutes, turning regularly. This timing will cook the meat to medium-rare, so adjust the cooking time if required. Remove the wallaby from the heat, wrap in foil and rest for 10 minutes.

To serve, thinly slice the wallaby fillet and arrange on a plate with the cherry chutney and a green salad, or with mash and veggies.

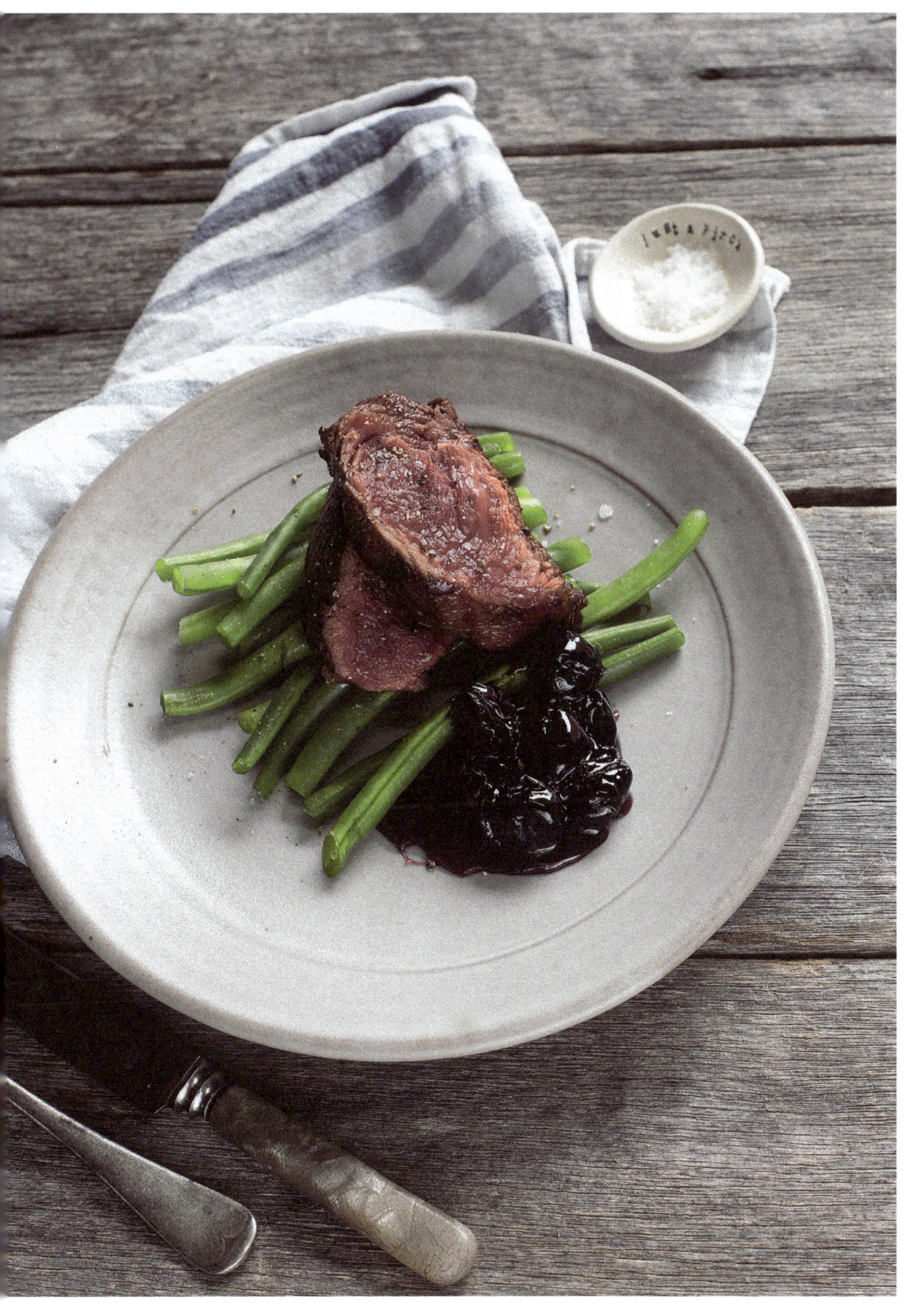

INDEX

A
Apple and Blackberry Pie 92
Apple Crumble 102
Apple Crumble Slice 104

B
Barbecued French toast with Bacon and Maple Syrup 34
Beef, Mushroom and Red Wine Pie 22
Black Forest Trifle 128
Blue Cheese, Pea and Prosciutto 136
Breakfast Bagel with Ricotta and Balsamic Tomatoes 54
Butter chicken and Naan Bread 114
Buttermilk Blinis with Superior Gold Smoked Salmon 148

C
Chili, Lemon and Garlic Squid Fettuccini 72
Creamy Crayfish Beef and Reef 74
Creamy Potato Salad 52
Crispy Baked Chicken Drumsticks 116
Crispy Pepper Berry Tassal Salmon with Ashbolt Sparkling Elderflower 164

D
Double Cooked King Island Beef in Stout with Potatoes and Gremolata 12

E
Easy Strawberry Jam 64

F
Fennel and Dill Crisp Coated Tuna with Lemon Aioli 78
Fermented Honey Garlic 56
Fermented Seeded Mustard 58
Fried Camembert Cheese with Strawberry and Lavender Coulis 134
Fried Sichuan Quail with Strawberry Chilli Sauce 118

G
Grilled Wallaby with a Roast Beetroot, Roast Garlic and Goats Cheese Tart 170

INDEX

H

Hazelnut and Rosemary Crusted Lamb Racks with Pinot Noir Butter Glaze 20
Hoi Sin Duck Breast with Beetroot Marmalade and Roasted Parsnips 120
Homemade Toffee Apples 90
Honey and Garlic Braised Farm Lamb Shanks with Pasta and Pumpkin 36
Honey Prawns 82
Huon Wood Roasted Salmon Frittata 156

I

Italian Amaretti Biscuits 112
Italian Pantry Meat Balls 16

K

Kahlua and Baileys Chocolate Tart 138
King Fish with Oyster Pâté in Pastry with Sweet Potato and Lemon Butter 84
King Island Baked Octopus 70

L

Lavender Salmon Gravlax with a Pickled Beetroot, Radish and Snow Pea Salad and Garlic Croutons 152
Lemon, Carrot and Polenta Cake With Lemon Syrup (Gluten Free) 96
Lemon Tart 98
Ling Burger with Pickled onion and cucumber 76

M

Minestrone Soup 32
Moroccan Inspired Goat Kebabs 28
Mushroom Pasta with Billy Goat Cheese 130

N

Nann Bread 114
Nashi Pear Tarte Tartin 106
Normandy Pork in Spreyton Fresh Cider with Apples, Celery and Walnuts 24

O

One Pot Salmon 146
Oysters with a Tangy Shallot Dressing 142

INDEX

P

Pan-fried Abalone with Spinach and Feta Salad 80

Petuna Ocean Trout with a Yoghurt Garlic Dressing and Pine Nut Topping 144

Pickled Octopus with a Greek Salad 86

Preserved Lemons 94

Pumpkin, Cauliflower and Red Lentil Dahl 66

Q

Quail with a Walnut, Blue Cheese and Apple Salad 122

Quince Paste 100

Quinoa, Broccoli and Sundried Tomato Salad 44

R

Ras al Hanout 28

Red Miso Huon Salmon 154

Rhubarb and Custard Tart 48

Rhubarb Clafoutis 126

Rib Eye with a Peppercorn, Pepper Berry, Lemon and Herb Rub and Lemon Button Mushrooms 14

Roast Tomato and Roast Garlic Soup 62

Rustic Country Kitchen Potato Bake 50

S

Seared Doo Town Wallaby with Beetroot Puree, Goat Cheese, and Spiced Balsamic Reduction 172

Slow Braised Lamb Shanks in Bruny Island Pinot Noir 18

Slow Cooked Duck 110

Slow Cooked Leap Farm Goat Shanks 30

Slow Cooked Rabbit with Fresh Pasta 168

Smoked Salmon and Fennel Salad 46

Spring Bay Mussels A la Brava 150

Spring Bay Mussels in a Tomato and Tarragon Broth with Saffron Aioli 160

Steamy Oriental Oysters 162

Summer Berry Pudding 60

Summer Vegetable and Salmon Pasta 158

INDEX

T
Thai Venison Salad 26
Tomato Sauce 42
Tongola Pea Pasta 132

V
Venison Carpaccio 38

W
Wallaby Fillet with Thyme Roasted Beetroot, Feta and Cherry Chutney 176
Wallaby Ragout 174

THANK YOU TO OUR GENEROUS SPONSORS

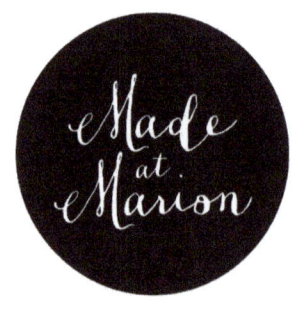

MADE AT MARION

Specialising in the delicate art of handmade pastries, Made at Marion uses fresh, local Tasmanian ingredients to produce luscious croissants, danishes and sourdough breads for the Bream Creek Farmers' Market. Baked fresh on the first Sunday of every month, Made at Marion serves up mouthwatering plain, almond and chocolate croissants, alongside escargot and kouigan amann to feed hungry Market goers and pastry connoisseurs. Got a sweet tooth? Follow the @madeatmarion Instagram account on Market morning to find what treats are available.

madeatmarion@gmail.com

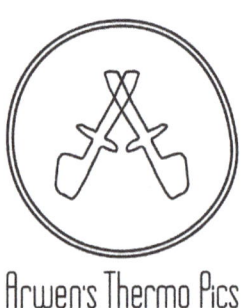

ARWEN'S THERMO PICS

Arwen is passionate about food. She loves cooking and experimenting with flavours and different cuisines from all around the world.

She gets a real buzz out of inspiring others to get the most out of their Thermomix. Arwen is a Qualified and experienced food photographer and stylist as well as cooking and organizing food shoots for other photographers. You can find the Thermomix versions of the recipes Arwen has submitted to this cookbook on her website and hundreds of other thermomix recipes arwensthermopics.com

Arwen Genge
Independent Thermomix Consultant Photographer
0400 145 977
arwen@arwensthermopics.com

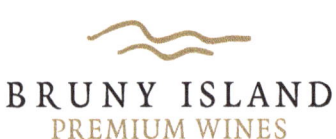

BRUNY ISLAND PREMIUM WINES

Carved from bush and pastureland on the outskirts of the sleepy little island settlement of Lunawanna on Bruny Island, is Australia's southernmost vineyard, Bruny Island Premium Wines.

We produce premium-quality, cool-climate wines, grown, harvested and crafted to reflect the regions terroir.

The Wine Bar & Grill serves all-day lunch in a relaxed alfresco dining area amongst the vines, featuring an extensive Bruny Island produce menu.

Bruny Island Premiere Wines is a family run business, that is passionate about providing customers with a unique enjoyable experience with a strong connection between premium, handcrafted wines, the island's fine produce, friendly welcoming hospitality and the beautiful, pristine, unspoilt environment.

0409 973 033
4391 Main Road Lunawanna Tasmania 7150
info@brunyislandwine.com
www.brunyislandwine.com

THANK YOU TO OUR GENEROUS SPONSORS

ENDLESS WAVES

Passionate Artistic Stylist dedicating Inspirational & Creative Hair.

We offer high quality Keune products & professional services in precision cutting & client analysis.

Keune Colour Expert, specialising in colour diversity & advanced techniques. We are highly trained and supported by The Keune Academy, which delivers extensive educational programs & events to stimulate creative minds.

Endless Waves hairdressing use and recommend Keune.

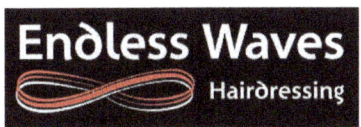

HUON AQUACULTURE

We've been farming Huon salmon in the pristine waters of Tasmania for over 30 years and in that time we've learnt a thing or two about the best way to raise the highest quality salmon in the world.

This focus on continual improvement and innovation in the way we farm has set the foundations for Huon Aquaculture to continue to grow sustainably into the future.

Peter & Frances Bender
(03) 6295 8111
huonaqua@huonaqua.com.au
PO Box 42, Dover, Tasmania 7117
www.huonaqua.com.au

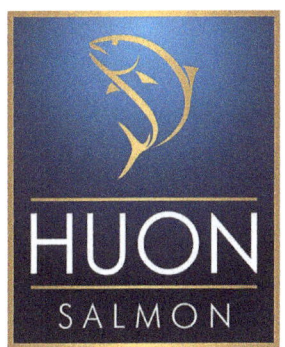

BANGOR

Bangor is a beautiful farming property managed for its stunning natural environment. Located on the Forestier Peninsula in Tasmania's south east, Bangor has over 35 km of breathtaking coastline and 5100 hectares of native forests, grasslands and wetlands. Over 2,100 hectares of Bangor are managed as conservation reserves, protecting a number of precious and iconic species including swift parrots, the wedge-tailed eagle, and the Tasmanian Devil. Bangor is also home to a 4 hectare vineyard, producing premium, award-winning cool-climate wine. Bangor's cellar door has a stunning view overlooking the vineyard, Blackman Bay, and the seaside township of Dunalley. Open 7 days, you can taste the full range of Bangor wines and enjoy a light meal made from local produce.

03 62 535 558
info@bangorshed.com.au
Bangor Shed, 20 Blackman Bay Road, Dunalley, Tasmania, 7177
www.bangorshed.com.au
Facebook: www.facebook.com/bangorshed
Instagram: @bangorshed

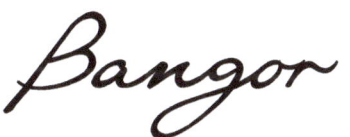

THANK YOU TO OUR GENEROUS SPONSORS

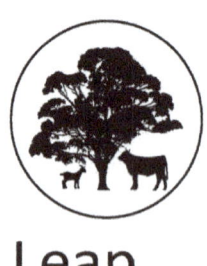

LEAP FARM

Leap Farm is a free-range goat and cattle farm in southeast Tasmania using organic principles to ensure sustainability and quality produce. Iain and Kate Field farm beef cattle, goats for meat and have a goat dairy herd. They ensure the animals have happy, healthy lives, which results in high quality produce, as sustainably as possible.

For more information, visit www. leapfarm.com.au

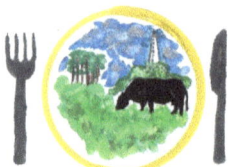

MEAT YOUR BEEF – KING ISLAND FARM TOURS

We are couple of "self – made" young farmers sharing our passion for farming and agricultural knowledge with you, through a guided visit of our beef farm on the north of King Island. King Island produces some of the best beef in the world and we will give you the opportunity to see it and taste with other local produce.

Walk the Walk Talk the Talk Eat the Beef

0427 118 903
3470 North Road, Egg Lagoon Tasmania 7256
ana@meatyourbeef-kingisland.com
www.meatyourbeef-kingisland.com

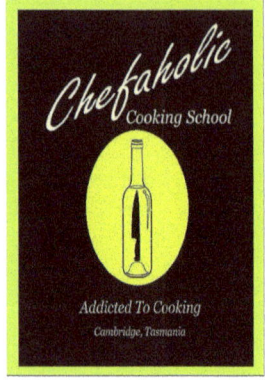

CHEFAHOLIC COOKING SCHOOL AND VINEYARD

Chefaholic Cooking School is situated at 8 Grapes Estate, a small Vineyard in Cambridge, Tasmania. It is a great passion realised for Stephen and his partner, Louise. Stephen's love of cooking and teaching come together in a rural, family setting, 15 mins from the centre of Hobart. Most produce is grown on site in the Veggie patch or supplied by local growers and businesses. The Cooking school is 100% Tasmanian family owned and funded and prides itself in supporting local Tasmanian businesses, farmers and growers.

Stephen and Louise create affordable, enjoyable and informative classes for small groups so Stephen may share his world class skills, and a few trade secrets along the way.

0407 175 720 or 0448 820 367
chefaholic.tas@gmail.com
www.facebook.com/chefaholic.cooking.school

THANK YOU TO OUR GENEROUS SPONSORS

TASSAL

Tassal salmon is so versatile it can be enjoyed by the whole family for breakfast, lunch or dinner. Proudly farmed in the cool Tasmanian waters, Tassal is committed to caring for the environment and producing healthy and sustainable salmon.

Visit www.tassal.com.au for more information.

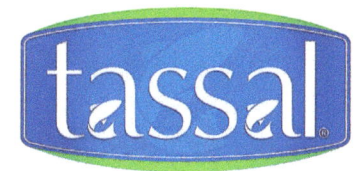

LUFRA HOTEL AND APARTMENTS

At our beautiful Eaglehawk Neck hotel, we're serving up our own special brand of hospitality, location and community. A short drive from Port Arthur and just an hour from Hobart International Airport, Lufra Hotel and Apartments is a breath of fresh, coastal air. Our hotel rooms and self-contained apartments offer quality accommodations with character and our on-site restaurant and café are charming, classic places to grab a bite to eat or throw a contemporary and elegant Eaglehawk Neck event or wedding reception.

03 6250 3262
reception@lufrahotel.com
380 Pirates Bay Drive, Eaglehawk Neck, 7179

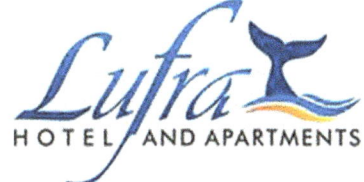

PORT ARTHUR LAVENDER FARM

Immerse yourself in one of nature's finest fragrances and explore the scent, taste and diversity that lavender Tasmania has to offer while enjoying the stunning Tasman Peninsula in the South East of Tasmania.

Nestled within seven hectares (18 acres) of lavender, rainforest and lakes and overlooking the ocean at Long Bay, Port Arthur Lavender's visitor centre and café showcase millennia-old uses of this fragrant flower alongside modern cuisine and a fully functioning essential oil distillery.

Stroll around the lavender trail or take in the ocean views while enjoying fresh Tasmanian produce in the lavender-inspired café.
Open 7 days (closed Christmas Day 25th December)

The lavender flowers are in their peak bloom from December through to February.

03 6250 3058
info@portarthurlavender.com.au
6555 Port Arthur Highway, Port Arthur Tasmania 7182

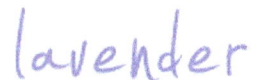

THANK YOU TO OUR GENEROUS SPONSORS

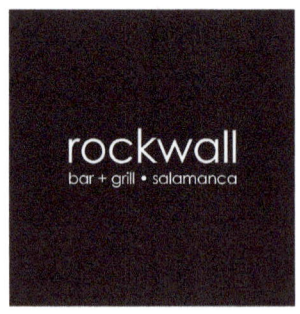

ROCKWALL BAR AND GRILL

Rockwall's cuisine encapsulates the state's reputation for four seasons in one day—oysters fresh from the waters off Bruny Island, Tasmanian salmon with crispy skin or pork loin rack, glazed with plum and tamarind on mash. Rockwall offers an extensive wine list and can match the dishes with wine available by the glass. You may even wish to try a cocktail.

03 6224 2929
89 Salamanca Place, Battery Point, Tasmania 7004
www.rockwallbarandgrill.com.au

PETUNA

Peter and Una Rockliff together with their families have spent many decades perfecting their artisan tasting products. Proudly Tasmanian, Petuna was established in 1949 when young professional fisherman Peter Rockliff met his future wife and business partner Una while docked at Bridport in Tasmania's north east. Together they would combine to create Tasmania's largest multi-species seafood business from their outlet in East Devonport. The now global business, with processing factory, smokehouse and value added processing facility, has been developed at the back of Una's original East Devonport retail outlet. Peter and Una's flagship retail store today has been transformed into 'Petuna Seafoods and Gourmet Pantry' – a seafood and gourmet heaven. Petuna also have a smaller retail seafood outlet at 253 Wellington Street in Launceston.

Peter & Una's work pioneering Ocean Trout and Atlantic Salmon in aquaculture has been recognised with an Order of Australia medal.

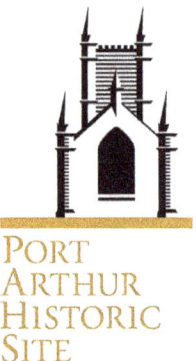

PORT ARTHUR HISTORIC SITE

The UNESCO World Heritage-listed Port Arthur Historic Site brings Australia's early convict history to life with world class interpretation, guided tours and dramatisations. A strikingly beautiful place with a harsh history, there is a lot to see and do with access to more than 30 historic buildings, a guided tour and harbour cruise included with your entry ticket.

1800 659 101 (Australia) +61 3 6251 2310 (International)
1800 659 202 (Australia) +61 3 6251 2311 (International)
reservations@portarthur.org.au
6973 Arthur Highway, Port Arthur, Tasmania
www.portarthur.org.au

THANK YOU TO OUR GENEROUS SPONSORS

TONGOLA GOAT PRODUCTS

Run by Iain and Kate Field, Tongola Goat Products is a small operation based in southeast Tasmania. This family enterprise is based on a small herd of Toggenburg goats (all individually named) that graze the paddocks and munch the blackberries. The milk from the ladies is kept on site and hand-crafted later in the day into cheese. Ensuring ethical and sustainable production is an important philosophy that underpins this business.

For more information, visit www.tongola.com.au

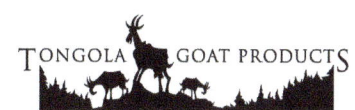

SPRING BAY SEAFOODS

"Spring Bay Mussels are Australian blue mussels (Mytilus galloprovincialis) carefully grown in the pristine deep cold waters off Tasmania's East Coast. Raised from babies in the company's novel bivalve hatchery the mussel spat are transferred to our marine farms and grow suspended on ropes and longlines for about 18 months. Mussels are prolific filter feeders surviving on micro-algae turning into one of Nature's peaches of the sea. Orange mussels are females – white mussels are males. Mussels take a few seconds to cook and can be enjoyed so many different ways.

03 6257 3614
info@springbayseafoods.com.au
488 Freestone Point Road, Triabunna, Tasmania, 7190

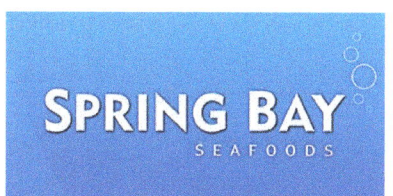

ASHBOLT

One of the reasons ASHBOLT products win awards is due to the way we grow our products

To nurture the soil, we use the clear clean water from the Derwent River and hundreds of tonnes of organic compost, seaweed fertilisers and nutrient-rich cover crops which we mulch back into tree rows.

Our unfinished goal is to drought-proof the farm, establishing efficient irrigation systems and shelter belts in each paddock and ultimately achieving a vibrant, relatively self-sufficient ecosystem.

We believe that the answer to the high quality and multi-medal winning status of our produce lies in the attention to detail and the particular 'terroir' (the interrelation between the trees, the terrain, the soil and its climate). Meet Anne at Salamanca Market

03 6261 2203
info@ashbolt.com.au
Glenora Rd, Plenty, Tasmania 7140

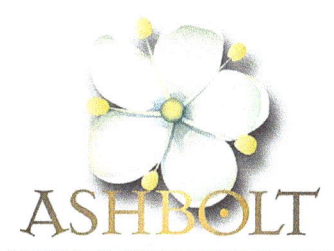

THANK YOU TO OUR GENEROUS SPONSORS

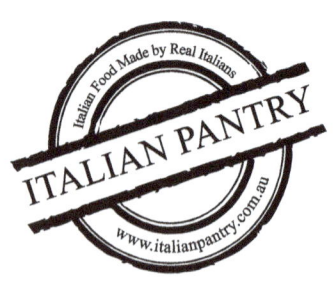

ITALIAN PANTRY

At the Italian Pantry the dining experience is akin to an Italian Trattoria. Along with our Italian Built wood fire pizza oven. the food is modest but plentiful, mostly following regional, local and family recipes.

An extensive and affordable regional wine menu with over 40 wines is available with many more on the reserve listing complementing an ever changing menu.

03 6231 2788
www.italianpantry.com.au
Retail/Deli Cafe/Restaurant 131-133 Murray Street Hobart
Cafe/Wholesale 27-29 Federal Street North Hobart

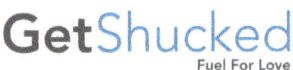

GET SHUCKED - BRUNY ISLAND OYSTERS

Get Shucked produces oysters of outstanding quality, sustainably cultivated in the pristine waters of Great Bay, Bruny Island, Tasmania.

We cultivate Pacific Oysters native to the pacific coast of Asia.

Our oysters are harvested daily and can be enjoyed at our fully licenced oyster bar overlooking our farm. We serve a range of Tasmanian wines, beers and ciders to go with our fresh or cooked oysters or swing by our drive through.

Suzanne Macefield
0439 303 597
1735 Main Rd Great Bay, Bruny Island, 7150

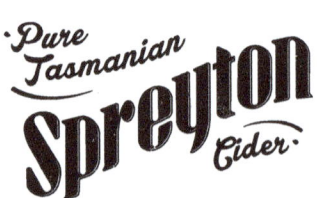

SPREYTON CIDER CO

Spreyton has been home to our families since the mid 1800's, and since 1908 we have been growing apples in this picturesque valley. For four generations we have grown the highest quality fruit for the people of Tasmania and the world.

When Spreyton Fresh (the parent of Spreyton Cider Co), was established in 1998 to begin making fresh apple juice, Spreyton also became synonymous with fantastic real apple juice that tasted like apples!

In 2011 it was time for the next step and Spreyton Fresh began experimenting with their first cider ferments and on the strength of those early experiments the Spreyton Cider Co. was launched. The company made the decision to keep the entire cider production process in house as that was the only way to ensure that our products would be made with the quality and integrity that is central to everything we do.

03 6427 3664
info@spreytonfresh.com.au
Cnr Melrose and Sheffield Roads, Spreyton Tasmania 7310

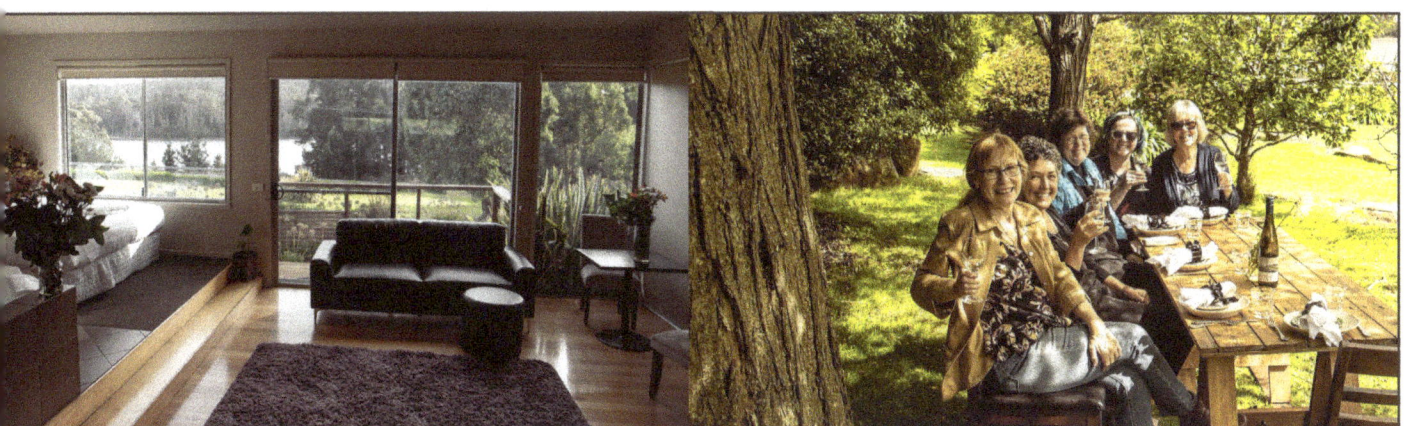

Little Norfolk Bay
EVENTS & CHALETS

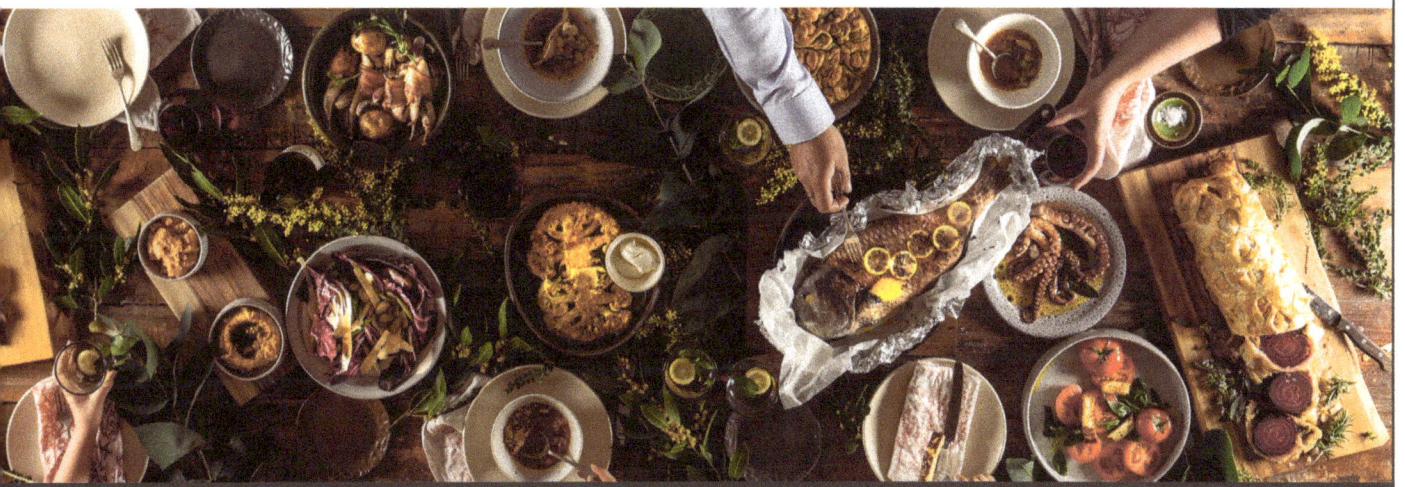

Accommodation, Cooking Retreats, Workshops and Indulgence Weekends in Taranna on the gorgeous Tasman Peninsula. Perfect for corporate or private gatherings and celebrations. Contact Chef and Host Eloise Emmett to design your unique experience.

www.eloiseemmett.com
www.littlenorfolkbayeventsandchalets.com

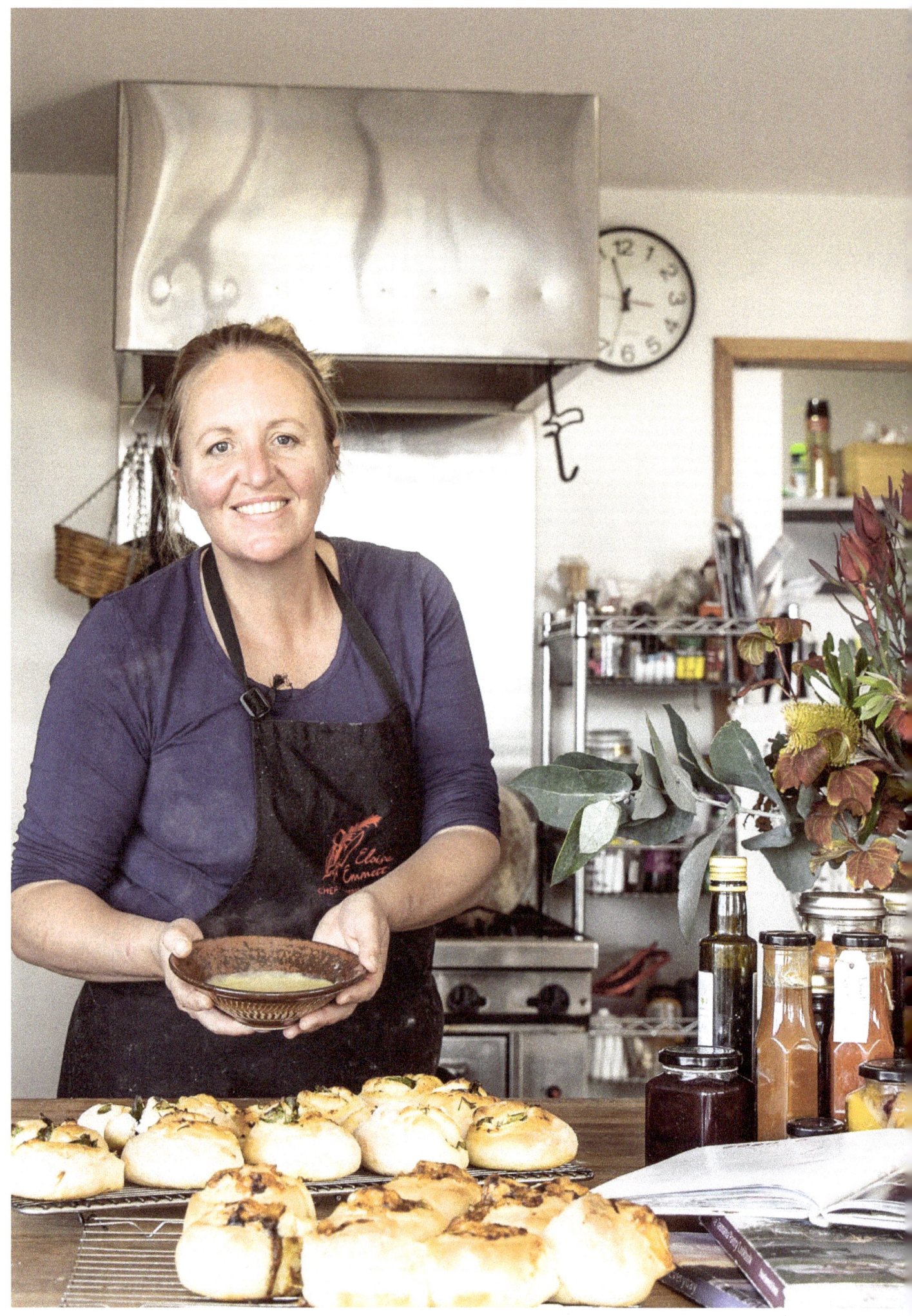

About the Author

Eloise Emmett is a Trade Qualified Chef with nearly 30 years experience in commercial kitchens, including 7 years as the Chef and owner of her own popular restaurant The Mussel Boys on the Tasman Peninsula. She now hosts weekend cooking retreats and indulgence weekends at Little Norfolk Bay Events and Chalets, which is a luxury accommodation retreat and boutique cooking school.

Eloise has been writing and photographing recipes for her popular website eloiseemmett.com since 2012. In 2013 Eloise co-authored the *Bream Creek Farmers Market Cookbook*, in 2015 she published *The Real Food for Kids Cookbook* and in 2016 she published the multi award winning *Seafood Everyday*. *Seafood Everyday* won **Best Fish and Seafood Book in Australia**, and **Best Book by a Woman Chef in Australia.** It then went on to become the third best seafood cookbook in the world, when it and won third place in **The Best Fish and Seafood** category at the **Gourmand World Cookbook Awards**. In 2017 Eloise published the first print of *The Tasmania Pantry* and in 2020 she published the second edition, *The Tasmania Pantry 2*.

Eloise loves cooking, styling and photographing food and shopping for props at op-shops and markets. She has three children and with her fisherman husband and they live on the stunning Tasman Peninsula in Tasmania. Most of all Eloise loves educating families about how important cooking, preparing meals and eating real food. Her core message, is that cooking is not hard and is a lot more economical way to feed your family, and she encourages even the busiest families to prepare easy meals from real food.

www.eloiseemmett.com

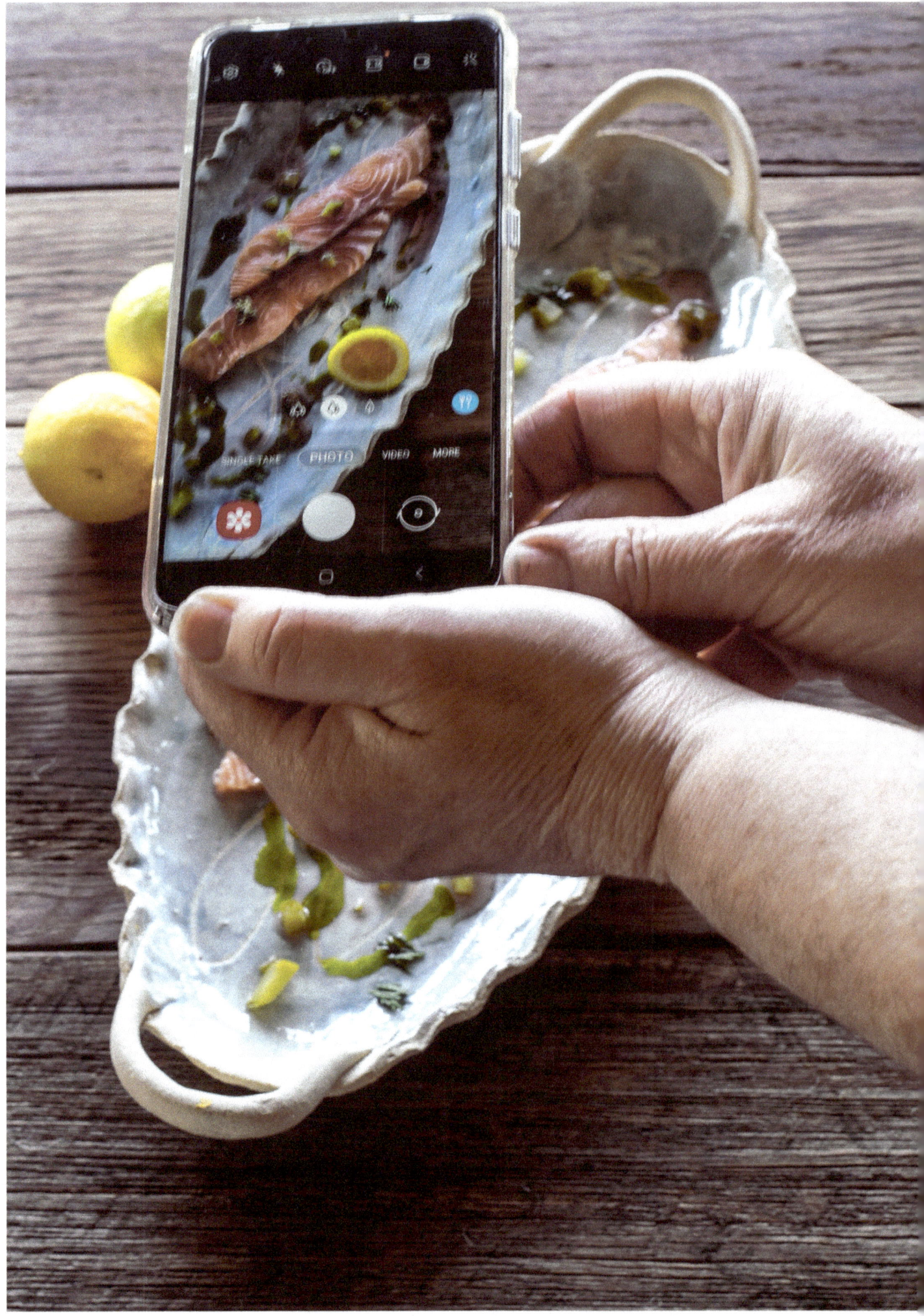

Feeling inspired?
Would you like to learn more?

You might enjoy my many in person and online workshops!

I cover many basics such as:

Seafood Cooking

Bread Making

Photography

Party Planning

Self Publishing

Phone Photography and Food Styling

Please find more information
at www.eloiseemmett.com

Eloise Emmett

CHEF   PHOTOGRAPHER   STYLIST

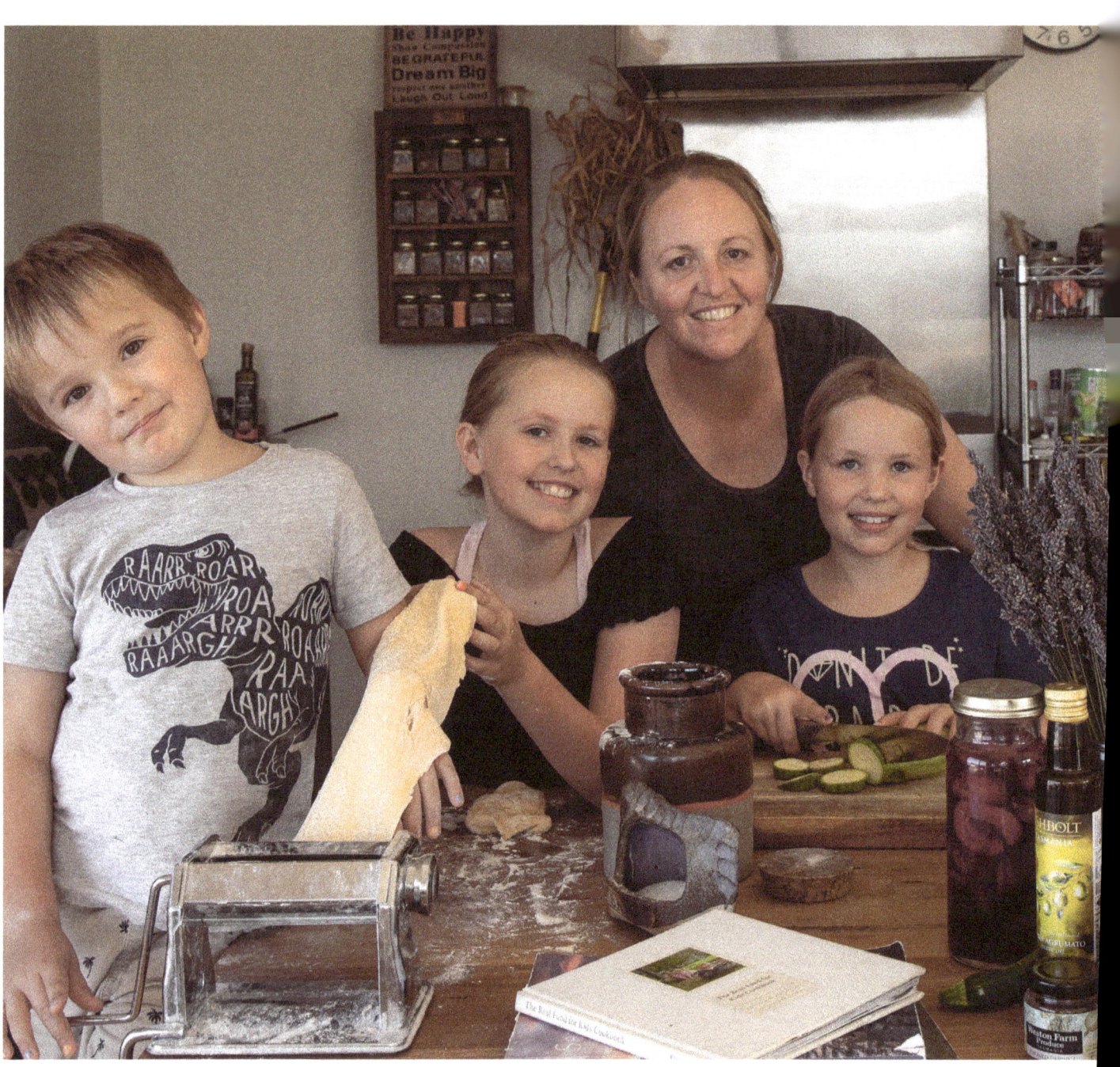

www.ingramcontent.com/pod-product-compliance
Lightning Source LLC
Chambersburg PA
CBHW041622020526
44118CB00052B/2994